Eating Vegan in Vegas

Eating Vegan in Vegas

in Vegas

Vegan City Guides

Edited by
Deborah Emin

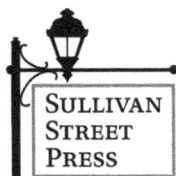

SULLIVAN
STREET
PRESS

Published by Sullivan Street Press, Inc., New York

Digital ISBN: 978-0-9963491-4-7
Print ISBN: 978-0-9976663-1-1

Contents

Preface

Eating Vegan in Vegas has become the first volume in a new travel series, as the original author of the *Eating Vegan in Vegas* blog, Paul Graham, had always intended it to become. By changing the focus of how we talk about being vegan, Sullivan Street Press is pleased to embark on this series that will eventually cover all of North America, whether by city or by region.

The world has changed in so many ways since I met Paul in 2012. At that time, his groundbreaking blog was one of the first to look at how Las Vegas, the most unlikely Vegan hub imaginable, had become so successful. Through discussions with Paul about turning his blog into a book, I also became a vegan.

Now the world's shifting has helped me take Paul Graham's idea to create a vegan city guide series and make it a reality. It is an honor to use Las Vegas as the first volume in the series.

As a frequent traveler, my wife and I have met lots of challenges while on the road. We have crisscrossed this country by train and by car. We camp out, we explore cities, we find ourselves in the middle of some very large states where there seem to be more acres of farmland than people, and in all these scenarios, we must eat.

What we have learned to do and what this travel series will help each traveler do is this: find the best, most appetizing food wherever you are. It is also necessary, as I see it, that we continue the bridge building no matter where we go.

For that reason, the series will focus on the points of interest that will be of particular interest to a vegan. For example, as you will see in the contents of this first volume, not all forty million yearly visitors to Las Vegas are interested in gambling.

For those who want to meet members of the animal rights community in Las Vegas, there is much to recommend in the chapter titled "The Ethics of Veganism," with its helpful links to ongoing activities. If you want to see what the state of vegan medicine is, an insightful chapter on that issue by Dr. Evan Allen is available ("Health"). There are also chapters on the vegan celebrities associated with Las Vegas ("Vegan Celebrities"), the cottage industries that have arisen from this focus ("It Takes a Village to Grow a Desert"), and the work of environmentalists in the state as well ("Desert to Food Hub").

We've also included in this volume what can be called a different introduction to Las Vegas, and while this book is for vegans, it does not only focus on food. The food is great, and I hope you'll enjoy as much of it as you have time for.

In honoring Paul Graham's foundational ideas about building bridges for a plant-based way of life, this series will celebrate the many ways this is occurring throughout North America.

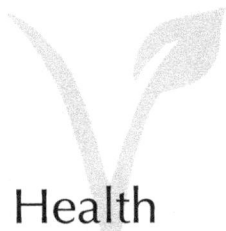

Health
Evan Allen, MD

In October 2011 in Las Vegas, shortly after my son was born, my wife brought me into our living room to watch a movie. I was a practicing, board-certified family physician, and this movie, *Forks over Knives*, purported to show how amazingly people could improve their health by eating a plant-based diet. I thought I was already eating plant based. I had been a vegetarian my whole life, never voluntarily eating any beef, chicken, seafood, fish, oysters, or pork. I told my friends that I wouldn't eat anything that had ever wiggled on its own. So I was skeptical about the film because I had recently had a physical and it showed that I had a fatty liver, even with my vegetarian diet.

Watching the film changed me. The information was astounding and had never been presented to me in the past, even during my medical training. I was surprised to see Dr. John McDougall in the film. I remembered him from my years at Pacific Union College in Angwin, California. During those years, I had worked as a phlebotomist at St. Helena Hospital and Health Center, where Dr. McDougall ran a program. While I had seen the patients and drawn their blood, I had known little about the actual workings of his program. It came as a surprise to watch him describe his patients' experiences in the film.

After watching the whole film, I became concerned because I thought patients would watch and come away with the idea that they could solve most of their chronic health problems simply by changing what they ate and drank. I certainly couldn't recall being tested on this material during my board exams, nor could I remember any questions about this in the weekly quizzes in my medical journals. Those exams and quizzes were mostly about pharmaceutical and surgical solutions to chronic problems.

Over the next few weeks, I began to research these findings. I expected to find lots of scientific data to support the position that modern medicine was doing the correct thing by focusing on drugs and surgery. What I found was almost the exact opposite. When there was scientific consensus, it was typically centered around the position of the film. Virtually every guideline that looked at diet in relation to disease recommended roughly the same thing: don't eat animal products (meat, seafood, dairy, eggs) and eat a diet that is almost entirely unrefined plant food.

After about a month, my wife and I decided to change how we ate.

During her pregnancy, she had put on seventy pounds and became what is called a gestational diabetic. Her blood pressure was dangerously high and went up to 200/100 after the delivery. When we changed how we ate, she lost all the weight within six months. Her blood pressure and blood sugar normalized.

I lost forty-five pounds over six months. Patients no longer recognized me. My asthma went away. I had chronic intestinal problems that were rapidly resolved. I was surprised at how much better I felt and at how much more energy and focus I had.

I decided to start making these dietary recommendations to patients. A few listened to what I had to say, and boy did they show me results!

Diabetics got off their medication. I had one patient who lost one hundred pounds in one year. Patients with intractable rashes got better. Sinus and allergy problems improved dramatically. But this advice only helped a small subset of my patients. Many heard my advice, but they either didn't or couldn't follow it due to their circumstances.

I decided to change my practice so I could achieve these dramatic results with a larger group of people.

One of the best things about living in Las Vegas is that it is a city that is friendly to people eating a plant-based diet. For us, however, the issue became more complicated because my wife suffers from severe migraine headaches that she gets when she consumes vegetable oils. For our health, and to keep her from getting migraines, we have to avoid foods that have vegetable oils in them. So while many of the restaurants that are available are great for people who want a plant-based meal, they didn't work well for us because of their use of these oils in most or all of their menu items.

Then we had a holiday party at a local restaurant, Panevino. Panevino is a gorgeous, five-star restaurant located just south of McCarran Airport.

My wife ordered her usual, noodles with just tomatoes and mushrooms with no oil and no oil-based sauce. The waiter took the order and went back to the kitchen while we waited.

As we were waiting for the food to come, a smartly dressed gentleman with an Italian accent approached us and asked politely why she had ordered the dish the way she had. She told her story, and it turned out that he ate the same way that we do. The man is Vincenzo Granata, and he is the general manager of the restaurant.

After further conversation, we realized that we had been at the same conference in plant-based eating about two months prior. Since then, my wife and I have been very lucky to be able to eat at Panevino whenever we want to have a dinner out without worrying about her getting a migraine.

Since opening Allen Wellness and Medical Center in 2014, my plant-based practice has grown rapidly. We have a staff nutrition coordinator and several tools we can use to do a dietary analysis of our patients. We have had remarkable successes. We offer concierge medical with either single-service pricing or annual memberships. We also offer classes each quarter with instruction on how to eat and prepare food to regain and maintain health.

Las Vegas is not the type of place where you would imagine it is easy to eat a healthy diet, but really it's a fantastic location for it.

There are Whole Foods Markets all over town, where you can always go to the food bar and get low-fat, healthy, vegan options. Several of the hotel chains also offer vegan menus, and there are a large number of ethnic restaurants that cater to the "no animal products or processed oils" crowd.

Another of our favorite places to go is Miko's Sushi on E. Windmill Lane. My son is in love with the miso soup there, and my wife and I love the vegan rolls. They have many options, but one of our favorites is the shiitake roll.

Many vegan options can be found at the restaurants at the Wynn and Encore hotels. Even though my wife can't consume any vegetable oils, we have had many fabulous meals there and the chefs have always been very accommodating. The hotels have a range of restaurants, from casual to fine dining and everything in between, so you can always find something that will work for you.

In addition, what I consider an added feature is that Las Vegas offers many great outdoor activities, hiking locations, and beautiful vistas. Red Rock Canyon is a gorgeous valley with rock walls of vibrant red ochre rimming the whole area. There are hiking opportunities for all ability levels. Valley of Fire State Park is about one hour out of town, and there you'll find the Rainbow Canyon, which you've already seen on television in car commercials but is worth the visit. Mount Charleston has stunning vistas and beautiful forests that experience snowfall in the winter. It's only thirty minutes out of town, making it possible to ski there in Lee Canyon.

Farther away, but within a day's journey, are the Grand Canyon in Arizona and Zion Canyon in Utah. Both are overwhelming natural wonders that you'll remember for a long time after seeing them. All of this activity will be healthy as well, and that is the point—to eat well and be active so we can live a good life. Ultimately, Las Vegas is a wonderful place to be for making healthy changes. I've dedicated the work I do at the Allen Wellness Center to making people happier and healthier.

When you are in Las Vegas and need medical care, please contact my office through our website (www.allenwellness.com) or you can call us at (702) 754-4900. I am a board-certified family physician and offer both membership and individual appointments in the wellness center. We have patients from all over the world and are happy to help with any acute or chronic condition you may have.

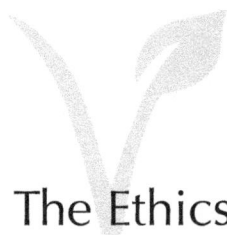

The Ethics of Veganism
William Bendik

The argument for choosing a vegan diet has three sides, or main reasons people make the change: health, environmental, and animal rights. Most people who become vegan are motivated by one or more of these concerns. As a scientist working in health care, I find the health and environmental benefits of eating vegan compelling and important to share. But in the six years since I went vegan, I've come to regard animal rights as the most significant aspect in a discussion of veganism, as preventing the harming and exploitation of animals can be the most emotionally and consciously rewarding aspect, often leading to a person's long-term commitment to a vegan way of life. It can be the hardest to quantify because it does not deal with lowered LDL values or with reduction in measured greenhouse gases. The only statistic that matters to vegans who are committed to the animals is the number that needlessly die or suffer each year for a system that is very much built to benefit businesses and exploit animals. For many, helping animals—doing all we can to reduce their suffering and deaths—is the heart of veganism, and these ethics represent a dividing line between eating a plant-based diet and being a vegan.

Making Progress

For many years, Las Vegas was a place with an appalling animal rights record, from the exploitation of animals for entertainment, to the prevalence of greedy, unethical backyard breeders and pet stores, to an overburdened animal shelter system that euthanized thousands of animals a year. Though there is still much work to be done, it is evident a shift is under way, and it is an exciting time in Las Vegas for animal rights advocates. Groups of organized vegans, animal rescuers, and other concerned members of the community are meeting and raising their voices around the Valley. They are joining forces to make our city a better one for the animals, and their efforts are paying off.

One such group, Vegas Veg, has been working to make a difference for animals in our community since 2007. Through their leafleting, tabling, and news rack programs, among other efforts, Vegas Veg does excellent educational work getting the population's attention and spreading the vegan message. They partner with many well-known organizations, such as Mercy for Animals, in their community outreach projects. They also host a Thanks-Living potluck event every year near Thanksgiving that is always filled with local vegans or those interested in learning more and an abundance of delicious vegan food.

Another group, Nevada Political Action for Animals, works on gathering support to elect animal-friendly officials and motivate the community to help pass ordinances and initiatives that directly impact the welfare of animals in the community. The work they do is progressive and crucial to creating lasting change in local law and representation for the animals.

There are numerous local animal rescue organizations all trying to rehabilitate and rehome unwanted animals, including the Nevada Society for the Prevention of Cruelty to Animals (SPCA), Heaven Can Wait Animal Society, Adopt a Rescue Pet, Hearts Alive Village, and many breed-specific rescue groups. Information on local animal recues, volunteer opportunities, and a wealth of information can be found at www.vegasanimalrescue.com. Las Vegas also has a dedicated group of TNR (trap, neuter, release) volunteers in the Community Cat Coalition of Clark County. They post volunteer positions on their website and are doing amazing work trying to keep our outdoor cat population down. The Las Vegas Valley Humane Society website features information on trapping cats as well as registering a feral (community) cat colony.

Creative Outlets for Vegans
There are a few local businesses and artists whose message aligns with veganism. One such artist is the one behind the Vegas-based movement known as Recycled Propaganda. Recycled Propaganda has a unique and creative approach to addressing a wide variety of social issues, including dietary concerns such as meat and sugar consumption. To me their most notable collaboration is with the VegeNation restaurant in downtown Las Vegas, where some thought-provoking art is always on display and a mural fills the back patio wall.

On the first Friday of each month, the Arts District in downtown Las Vegas is host to dozens of artists and food vendors, some of which provide vegan offerings or a full vegan menu. It is there that a few of the local vegan popup food vendors started businesses before local farmers' markets grew more successful.

Farmers' markets have multiplied throughout the Valley over the last few years, and many vegan or incidentally vegan food and products can be found there, as well as local artists and entertainers and family-friendly activities. Here is a listing of current local farmers' markets:

Bruce Trent Park Farmers' Market
Wednesdays, 4 p.m.–8 p.m.
(Rampart and Vegas Drive)

Country Fresh Farmers' Market
Downtown Henderson in the Water Street Events Plaza
Thursdays, 9 a.m.–4 p.m.

Henderson Pavilion
Fridays, 10 a.m.–4 p.m.

The District Farmers' Market
Thursdays, 4 p.m.–8 p.m.; March–June and September–December

Downtown 3rd Farmers' Market
Fridays, 9 a.m.–3 p.m.

Downtown Summerlin Farmer's Market
Saturdays, 9 a.m.–2 p.m. under the Pavilion

fresh52 Farmers and Artisan Market
Tivoli Village
Saturdays, 9 a.m.–2 p.m.

Sansone Park Place
Sundays, 8:30 a.m.–1 p.m.

The Green Chefs Farmers' Market at the Springs Preserve
Thursdays, 10 a.m.–3 p.m.

Las Vegas Farmers' Market at Floyd Lamb State Park
Saturdays, 10 a.m.–2 p.m.; mid-March–mid-December

Gardens Park in Summerlin
Tuesdays, 4 p.m.–8 p.m.; mid-March–mid-December

Feed Your Spirit

When I think about what is moving the spirit of veganism in Las Vegas, I think of The Reset Project, which brings local leaders in health and wellness together with the community to achieve a healthier lifestyle by resetting the mind, body, and spirit. Their signature event occurs on the first Sunday of each month in downtown Las Vegas and features a variety of speakers, wellness activities, a spiritual session, and personal growth tips. Typically the morning ends with participants sharing a delicious vegan meal.

Another center of spirituality and community focus is Govinda's Center of Vedic India. Located on Dean Martin Drive, it is very close to the Las Vegas Strip and the center of the Vegas Valley. They hold yoga classes, have a gift shop, and provide a low-cost vegetarian and vegan buffet, and even a free buffet on Sundays. Call ahead to find out which of the many services are available, as there are various events they might be holding on any given day of the week.

One organization spreading a message of compassion while also helping people in need is the Las Vegas branch of Food Not Bombs. This group meets at Huntridge Park on Sundays and Mondays and distributes vegetarian and vegan food that would otherwise go to waste to anyone looking for a meal. They are always looking for donations and assistance in the good work they do.

Just a scenic three-and-a-half-hour drive from Las Vegas is one of my favorite places to renew my spirit. Best Friends Animal Sanctuary is located in Kanab, Utah, close to Zion National Park, and is a haven for those who want to see animals being treated with the care and respect they deserve. Best Friends is nationally known for their no-kill and anti-puppy-mill initiatives. The Animal Sanctuary has an excellent tour and volunteer program, and many of the staff members will go out of their way to tell you about the animals they have worked so hard to care for. There are pet-friendly cabins and cottages you can rent to stay in, as well as RV sites. Against the gorgeous backdrop of Angel Canyon and the stunning red bluffs of Utah's steppes and hills, you will get the opportunity to see horses, pigs, goats, rabbits, cats, and dogs, all living the best lives possible, and many seeking forever homes. Don't forget to visit the gift shop, and make sure you are able to attend lunch at the café. Five dollars buys some of the freshest and most tasty vegan food that can be found for miles around (although Kanab has some great veg-friendly dining and even a vegan grocery store!).

Las Vegas is home to its own nonprofit animal sanctuary that is actively working to create a safe haven for animals in need. The ONE Family Animal Sanctuary facility is not currently open to the public, but they share their work on their Facebook page and accept donations for the care of their animals.

Special Events

Health, Healing, and Happiness is a yearly event in Las Vegas put on by Belsandia. The two-day program features well-known vegan speakers and authors such as Dr. Michael Greger, Dr. John McDougall, Dr. Joel Fuhrman, Robert Cheeke, and Chef A. J. There are always varied and interesting presentations and vendors, and the event also offers yoga and fitness classes. The next Health, Healing, and Happiness event will be held on June 10–12, 2016, at the Tuscany Suites.

Vegas VegFest is happening on April 9, 2016. It will be held at the Clark County Government Center and has already generated a lot of interest in the local community, as well as with those looking to travel to Vegas for its first-ever VegFest. Announced speakers so far are Paul Shapiro from the Humane Society and the Vegan Bros. The event will be put on by an all-volunteer base and is coproduced by Compassion Works International. It is free to everyone, but they will be accepting donations. There are already some great local businesses announced as food vendors, including Mint Indian Bistro and VegeNation.

The Movement Advances

As a result of the work so many caring citizens are doing in the community, encouraging changes have occurred that will help the Valley's animal population. In 2009, the City of Las Vegas passed a mandatory spay and neuter law, a basic measure and first step toward preventing the suffering and deaths of so many animals.

In September of 2013, the Las Vegas Zoo closed. Controversy surrounded this local landmark, as it was often the feature of many high-profile media stories involving the conditions the animals were kept in. Anyone who has endured a Vegas summer outside knows that this climate is only fit for the very heartiest of creatures. The zoo's closure appeared to reflect a small change in public attitude—a beginning to the end of the old way of doing things.

The current energy toward animal welfare in Las Vegas is positive and hopeful. During the course of writing this chapter, the Las Vegas City Council passed an ordinance requiring local pet stores to work with local rescue organizations for their supply of animals within two years, banning them from purchasing pets through out-of-state puppy mills. I was fortunate to be present during the council meeting and was able to be one of dozens of local residents who stood before the mayor and council members and presented our reasons the ordinance should be passed. It was invigorating as someone who supports and believes in animal rights to see so many other like-minded people take time to come and speak on behalf of the voiceless. Many of the people waited patiently for hours as the council worked through the other matters on their agenda, and when the time came to speak, everyone did so passionately and articulately. The issue was controversial because there are technically only two pet shops left in the city selling dogs, cats, and piglets. Yet the ordinance being passed was an important step and again sets the tone that our community is fed up with the neglect and disposable attitudes that the general populace seems to regard animals with, as well as allowing the senseless euthanasia of so many healthy animals each year to continue.

Shortly after the pet store ordinance passed, The Animal Foundation, which operates the city's largest animal shelter, held a press conference announcing a strategic plan to decrease the number of animals killed at the shelter and achieve a 90 percent "save rate" by the end of 2020. The shelter currently takes in around ninety animals per day. The plan includes creating and expanding lifesaving programs, such as a trap-and-release program for free-roaming cats; upgrading the facility's medical capabilities; and renovating and adding to the existing shelter. They also called for the community to support their efforts, which will be necessary to achieve these goals.

If people will not take the time to make informed and responsible decisions, and businesses exploit that ignorance regarding animals, then someone needs to be their voice and say enough is enough. It is through these continued efforts that progress can be made, that the public can be educated, and that animal welfare can be ensured. If you ever have the opportunity to do anything, however big or small, to be a voice for the animals and represent your own unique viewpoint, I encourage you to do so! It may renew your conviction and leave you a proud member of your community, as it did for me.

Links

Adopt a Rescue Pet
http://www.adoptarescuepet.vegas

The Animal Foundation
http://animalfoundation.com

Best Friends Animal Society
http://bestfriends.org

Community Cat Coalition of Clark County
http://www.c5-tnr.org

Compassion Works International
http://www.cwint.org

Food Not Bombs Las Vegas
http://foodnotbombslasvegas.org

Govinda's Center
http://govindascenter.com/home.html

Health, Healing, and Happiness
http://www.health-healing-happiness.com

Hearts Alive Village
http://www.havlv.com

Las Vegas Valley Humane Society
http://www.lvvhumane.org

Recycled Propaganda
http://recycledpropaganda.com

The Reset Project
https://www.facebook.com/theresetproject/?fref=ts

Vegas Veg
http://www.vegasveg.org

Vegas VegFest
http://www.vegasvegfest.com

Desert to Food Hub
Mary Beth Horiai

Las Vegas sits on the floor of the Mojave Desert and the landscape is arid and rocky—certainly not conducive to farming and agriculture. The challenges Southern Nevada faces for growing food are many: hard and dry soils, limited water, and extremely hot temperatures. Because of these challenges, Las Vegas has grown to depend on imported food via plane delivery and primarily via one key highway.

This chapter will take a brief look at the history of food in Las Vegas and the challenges facing food production in Southern Nevada. Next we will examine the catalysts that are contributing to a more a sustainable food movement and the people and organizations behind the movement. Finally, I'll give you a look at the organizations supporting this movement toward making Las Vegas a self-sustaining food hub.

Everyone knows Las Vegas, therefore many refer to it even when they may be discussing nearby areas such as Henderson, North Las Vegas, Clark County, or even Pahrump and Boulder City. These areas in Southern Nevada are often forgivably referred to as Las Vegas even when they mean a different location. For our purposes, I too will just call this section of Southern Nevada, Las Vegas.

Vegas Lifeline

Interstate 15, the corridor that's for all transport into and out of Las Vegas, was severely affected by the forest fires in 2015 in California. Cars and trucks caught on fire, which ended up melting the roads. The highway had to be closed, blocking the passage of visitors and food from Southern California to Southern Nevada.

Unlike any other city in the United States, Las Vegas must not only feed its two million residents but has more than forty million visitors coming per year. Over $300 million worth of fruits and vegetables are imported along this vital highway every year. When transportation stops, so does food delivery.

In 2001, Las Vegas, like elsewhere in the United States, saw businesses stopped cold immediately after September 11. The town suffered an economic shock not having a constant flow of planes flying in, packed with visitors ready to deposit their funds into the dependent infrastructure. However, even more shocking was the realization that when transportation stops, so does food delivery.

Sometimes it takes a disaster for a city to realize how dependent it is on systems that it does not control. While the desert may be a landscape of parched earth and low rainfall, prior to this realization that 95 percent of its fresh fruits and vegetables had to be imported, there were those in Las Vegas who also realized that a paradigm shift had to be made in order for the city and the region to survive. Too many hazards exist: fires, floods, and melted tarmac pose potential hazards to the safe and steady delivery of these vital products.

History and Challenges

When it comes to food in Las Vegas, people often think of endless cheap buffets or, more recently, lavish, high-end restaurants with star chefs at every location. The Las Vegas Valley, however, came from more humble beginnings. Despite the arid desert climate, early Native American tribes like the Paiutes lived off of roots, cacti, pine nuts, and indigenous wildlife. They shared some of their techniques for hunting and gathering with the early Mormon settlers.

Over the last century, Las Vegas's landscape has expanded from the Strip outward in all directions. New developments have filled in the prized spaces closest to the Strip. Southern Nevada has never been thought of as an agricultural hub; however, there are several dozen farms in Las Vegas and the surrounding areas, as well as more than two dozen community gardens.

As the population of Southern Nevada grows and the tourist industry continues to thrive, so does the demand for food.

Transportation struggles, flight cancelations, gas prices, droughts, and food pricing spikes all contribute to food insecurity for this desert oasis.

Catalysts

Like a young adult leaving the comfort of home to venture out to become self-supporting, Las Vegas and the surrounding communities have started the journey toward food sustainability.

There are many catalysts steering this food movement forward. One catalyst is the widespread awareness of the connection between diet and health, particularly the rise in heart disease, obesity, cancer, and type 2 diabetes, especially in children. According to the Center for Disease Control, one-third of premature deaths in the United States are attributed to poor nutrition. Child obesity in Southern Nevada is a concern and has spurred on nonprofit organizations such as Create a Change Now and Green Our Planet to assist schools in bringing an awareness of the relationship among food, health, and test scores to the educators.

Contrarily, the legalization of medical cannabis has also stimulated the growth of many cottage industries such as businesses selling LED grow lights, hydroponic equipment, and soil nutrients. The increase of marijuana agriculture goes hand in hand with finding new, inventive ways to successfully grow plants in a desert environment.

Climate change, leading to regional droughts and crop reductions, is the overriding catalyst for communities to start more local, sustainable, and indoor food production. As food shortages increase, so do food prices. Food insecurity by either physical or economic circumstances essentially affects everyone, but especially those living in a desert.

What Grows in Vegas Stays in Vegas: People behind the Movement

Las Vegas is known for being a place where entrepreneurs and risk takers can place their bets. The massive tour industry has turned Las Vegas into the entertainment capital of the world. Over the last decade, the solar industry has moved quickly into Southern Nevada and made great strides. And more recently, leaders in a variety of specialties have integrated together on many projects revolving around the support of local, sustainable, grassroots food production.

In October of 2015, the Nevada Chapter of the U.S. Green Building Council (USGBC) hosted the first Green School STEM Summit for more than three hundred teachers and local leaders. It was a collaborative effort from fourteen community organizations and three school districts. One of the goals of the summit was to spur more STEM learning through gardens in schools.

The Green Schools Summit was successfully spearheaded by the president of USGBC, Rick Van Diepen. Van Diepen claims that it has been hard to convince partners of the need to improve their resiliency. He demonstrates that despite the challenges of an arid climate, other regions such as Israel and Australia are successfully producing sustainable food. Van Diepen is encouraged by the enthusiasm and drive of others he is collaborating with.

Rick Passo, a man that has his hands in all things green and food related in Las Vegas, is Van Diepen's most passionate collaborator. They have been nicknamed Team Rick, and there is no stopping them.

Green Our Planet, a nonprofit responsible for a steady momentum of new school gardens in the Clark County School District, has helped find funding and farmer support for school gardens. The education of young students and teachers through a garden covers many aspects of science, health, math, nutrition, and teamwork. Through regular visits and training from the farmers of Garden Farms of Nevada, the schools have been able to see not only better test scores but also an increase in the students' vegetable intake. Numerous studies support this and show that having a school garden can raise students' test scores, increase environmental awareness, and combat the obesity epidemic. Just like Ron Finley, a guerilla gardener from South Central LA, says, "If kids grow kale, kids eat kale." Green Our Planet has witnessed these results firsthand at more than seventy-five school gardens they helped build in just four short years.

Tiffany Whisenant, the manager at Garden Farms of Nevada, reminisces about just a few short years ago when many community leaders gathered together for "green jelly meetings" to throw around ideas and find solutions for the many food challenges in Las Vegas. Those discussions turned into organizing some of the many social media groups discussed in the next chapter and the planning of community garden steering committees, and it has grown from there.

Garden Farms of Nevada began when the founders, Brian and Brittany, decided that they wanted to share the talents they had developed from growing their own food for many years. They worked with homes, schools, restaurants, hotels, apartment complexes, and even senior centers.

They helped build raised-bed gardens and sunken gardens and taught canning, planting, and composting methods, as well as landscaping—all in a sustainable manner. Check out the gardens they helped create at the Element Hotel in Summerlin, the

Cancun community garden on the Strip, and the Paradise Square apartments on Tropicana and Eastern.

Longtime resident Steve Rypka has seen the levels of advocacy rise over the years, but Rypka reluctantly admitted it has been hard at times to stay in Las Vegas. He says, "For many years I wanted to escape from a city that didn't have an infrastructure of sustainable values." He has come to see Las Vegas as a perfect place to make change happen. He has mentioned people like author Paul Graham promoting vegan lifestyles, Team Rick bringing a strong coalition of people together to create a food hub, Ciara Byrne and the Green Our Planet crew making school gardens happen, and Rypka's own doctor, Evan Allen (see the chapter titled "Health"), giving educational seminars on vegan health to Southern Nevadans.

Innovative Food Hub and Other Solutions

What is a food hub? It is a business incubator for farmers and producers that can sell value-added products. Even more so, a food hub for Las Vegas needs to address food independence and food inequality. Las Vegas has the perfect market to sell fresh, healthy, organic produce that restaurants can boast about. Coupling this with the need to also provide nutritious food for the underserved communities gives Las Vegas the opportunity to provide a wide range of fruits and vegetables to feed the growing population in Las Vegas.

As we look to the future, reports on NPR discussed a possible food hub joining a massive development in Northern Las Vegas where a new electric car company, Faraday Future, is scheduled to open in the near future. There is talk that Tony Hsieh's Airstream park, which some refer to as an "urban camping area," is an ideal place for a food hub. Others, like Tiffany, are working toward multiple food hubs organically rising up in the many food deserts around the Valley.

However, the most solid plans are being made by Team Rick. They are in talks with Kerry Clasby, the "Intuitive Forager," an amazing farmers' market advocate. Kerry travels the length of California and Oregon in search of first-rate produce that she markets to the high-end restaurants on the Strip.

Presently, after the fresh52 markets on Saturdays in Summerlin at Tivoli Village and on Sunday in Henderson at Sansone Park finish, they donate their unsold produce to charities. Charities like Project Angel Face and Three Square receive hundreds of pounds a week to feed the underprivileged. These markets also house several vegan vendors such as Grass Roots, Virgin Cheese, Bite, Garden Grill, and Bloomin' Herbs.

Team Rick and Kerry Clasby have also made connections with the Nevada Food Council, the Las Vegas Global Economic Alliance, the Downtown Project, and Ken McCowan, former director of the Design Department at the University of Nevada, Las Vegas (UNLV). McCowan led research that created a sustainability atlas for the city of Las Vegas, identifying food resources and food deserts.

Together this team is determined not only to create a food hub for local, urban, and indoor grown food, but also to create a social machine that allows high-end resorts to work together with farmers and organizers that also serve the communities and those in need. After much research, McCowan sees Las Vegas as a bellwether and has hope for a robust vision of a food hub.

Team Rick was also responsible for bringing Steve Ritz, from the Green Bronx Machine, to Las Vegas to be the keynote speaker at the Green Schools Summit. Ritz has a famous charged-up TED talk and was recently featured in the PBS documentary *In Defense of Food* by Michael Pollan. Ritz has turned schools in the Bronx into a green paradise. His programs have helped raise test scores in at-risk schools and dramatically improve the health of the students and the neighborhood. His goal at Green Bronx Machine is to show everyone *we can grow, reuse, resource, and recycle our way into new and healthy ways of living.*

What does Ritz have to do with Las Vegas? Through the community excitement he witnessed and his connections with Team Rick, he has agreed to come to Las Vegas to open a wellness education center to teach vocational training around food production for at-risk schools in Las Vegas.

All the pieces are coming together for a major downtown food hub; for possibly an indoor food hub adjacent to Faraday Future in Northern Las Vegas; or even, as Tiffany from Garden Farms hopes, for smaller area food hubs that start and grow organically. However it begins, Las Vegas now has all the parts: a group of motivated individuals and organizations; a full-range market with high-end restaurants wanting a more stable, locally grown source; and a social element of being able to feed the communities in Las Vegas, especially the lower income areas with greater need for healthier, affordable fresh produce.

The Future Is Now

The near future of healthy, plant-based food security in Las Vegas is ultimately dependent on the grassroots efforts of people. Las Vegas has the advantage of attracting people from everywhere for myriad reasons. There are many Las Vegas vegans with claims to having been born here, yet most of us are transplants from other cities, states, and countries. While doing research for this chapter, I was able to talk to many people with invaluable information and enthusiasm. While there are multitudes of smart, passionate proponents of local, sustainable food production, it was impossible not to come in contact with one key advocate, Rick Passo. No matter who I spoke to, they would end the conversation with "you should speak to Rick Passo."

Luckily for me, I did it in reverse. Passo was one of my first calls and led me to most of the individuals and organizations previously mentioned. Passo's prediction of the future is the future is now. "Food cuts across all boundaries: cultural, religious, and language," says Passo.

Las Vegas is more than ready to move forward to either organically create small food hubs around communities, as is Tiffany's hope, or, as Rick Van Diepen believes, to take advantage of the engine that is Las Vegas with its unending demands. A once discouraged Rypka claims that "Vegas is the perfect place to make a change happen."

A transformation of Southern Nevada's food system is an opportunity to inspire many to healthier, smarter, plant-based lifestyles.

Links

CCSD Obesity Research
https://www.southernnevadahealthdistrict.org/download/stats
-reports/ccsd-height-weight-report-2013.pdf

Community Gardens
http://beta.allrise.co/a/0770db3d4933a66f/Community-Gardens
-remain-an-excellent-example-of-Grassroots-Sustainability-in-action
-for-Las-Vegas-Henderson-North-Las

Farmers' markets
http://beta.allrise.co/a/07708b8749323285/Farmers-Markets-in
-Clark-County-including-Las-Vegas-Henderson-North-Las-Vegas
-Boulder-City-and-Pahrump

Farms
http://beta.allrise.co/a/07708cf349322ff1/Commercial-Farms-in
-Clark-County-including-Las-Vegas-Henderson-North-Las-Vegas
-Boulder-City-Pahrump

It Takes a Village to Grow a Desert
Mary Beth Horiai

As a result of the unanticipated and welcomed growth in local food production, consequent growth in supportive industries and organizations has, in turn, spurred more growth. These cottage industries have integrated nicely to form a supportive web in order for community gardens to develop, for school gardens to come together, and for the dream of food hubs to be realized. The passionate people behind these organizations are small in number, and many times you will meet the same people belonging to or spearheading several enterprises; nonetheless, the fervor is catching on.

Just like a plant needs sunshine, water, minerals, and care to grow, so does a food movement. While Vegas has plenty of sunshine and plenty of land, the desert is a challenging prospect for growing food. Regardless of its challenges, Southern Nevada is forging ahead toward creating healthier and more sustainable food security. This could only be done with the actions of supportive entrepreneurs that have opened businesses selling more water-efficient soils, alternative indoor farming technologies, and seeds and seedlings that grow well under our desert conditions. In addition to businesses, inventive nonprofits that cooperate with other organizations continue to find niches to fill and work hand-in-hand with farmers, educators, chefs, and corporate sponsors.

In the following pages, we will first look at some soil alternatives and innovative plans for seed exchanges. Next we will lay out the variety of alternative farming and gardening methods being employed in the Las Vegas Valley. Finally we will present innovative ideas of things to do while visiting Las Vegas surrounding plant-based food communities, as well as events and meet-up groups.

From the Ground Up: Challenges of Soil and Seeds

Most Las Vegans, including myself, have had a hard time growing things in their yards. This is mainly due to caliche, a layer where soil particles are cemented together by lime that blocks drainage. Most soil needs lots of added enrichments.

The University of Nevada Cooperative Extension has a lifelong learning campus located just south of the McCarran Airport. There are 270 master gardeners in Southern Nevada that have gone through a seventy-hour training course. Upon completion, they volunteer their time on various local projects, teach seminars, and answer gardening questions on their hotline. There they teach and assist with ways to change or enrich your soil, ideas for composting, and guidance on what plants grow best in the desert. If you visit on a Friday, the master gardeners give free tours of the Demonstration Gardens. All master gardeners are fully qualified, but if you can, ask for Rich, who is happily retired and will give you information on anything you need to know.

One soil solution comes from an innovative local start-up called Wonder Soil. I met the owner of Wonder Soil, Patti, at a fundraiser for the Green Schools Summit. She was so excited to show me how her compressed, dry soil expanded by adding a small amount of water. The pellets of soil reminded me of those snake fireworks we used to light on the Fourth of July. The pellets are made mostly from coconut core, which allows for faster germination and uses 50 percent less water. Her enthusiasm was so catchy that I agreed to come visit her factory near the Las Vegas Strip.

Wonder Soil, like many other cottage industries commencing in the last couple of years, has done more than just sell their product. They have integrated their product with the waste from resort hotels such as the MGM and the Cosmopolitan. By collecting organic waste from the hotel kitchens, they are able to close the loop by dehydrating and sterilizing the biomass in a contraption called an Eco-bin, thus creating more soil compounds to add to the pellets. Patti is more than happy to give visitors a tour of the plant, which is conveniently located just off of Las Vegas Boulevard.

Seeds of Change

Many of the organizations that are building school gardens in the Clark County School District encounter challenges in obtaining trustworthy seeds. They often have to depend on investigative blogs to find out where to purchase non-GMO seeds. One diligent teacher, Jennifer Davis, from Desert Oasis High School, recommends Johnny's Seeds in Maine and Territorial Seeds in Oregon; both have convenient online ordering. Davis started the first high school garden maintained by three hundred special needs students and their teachers. Since starting the garden, they now teach the students how to save their seeds to use for the next harvest.

Despite the lack of local seed distributors, there are still many other creative schemes under way in Las Vegas. The Green Valley Library in Henderson has taken to heart the idea of sharing seeds. In the spring of 2015, they partnered with the nonprofit Great Basin Permaculture and installed an old-fashioned gum ball machine. Upon entering the library, you can pop a quarter in the machine and get a surprise package of seeds. These seeds were from a variety of forty different herbs, vegetables, and flowers that are local and native to the area. This machine was coupled with a miniprogram where would-be gardeners could learn how to save seeds from their summer crops, and then in the fall, the library would host a community seed swap. They are inviting people to eventually bring back their seeds.

Ideally, the seed library could mimic a book library, where the seeds are common goods borrowed and returned for others to share. According to Kevin Scanlon, the library's head of adult services, the Green Valley Library is the first to become a lending library of seeds as well as books. The Green Valley Library will be partnering with the state of Nevada to help track the genomes of the seeds. They are continuing to offer programs for kids and teens to learn more about various aspects of gardening.

Hopefully other libraries in the Valley could follow this pilot program. Residents could check out seeds just like they would check out books, only for a bit longer period of time. The exchange would be a promise on the honor system, to return the next generation seeds back into the library for others to check out. There are many details that still need to be worked out, but certainly libraries in the digital age are in need of new ideas to draw people in.

Alternative Farming

The many alternatives to traditional farming include urban raised beds, indoor and vertical agriculture, and a variety of hydroponics. All of these are being successfully put into use in Southern Nevada. Many of the home and school gardens talked about in the previous chapter are using raised beds in order to control the soil contents.

Hydroponics, a nonsoil technology that uses primarily water, is also very popular. Some companies started their businesses in hopes of a cannabis bump. One hydroponic owner, selling grow lights, soil, and fertilizers, told me that sales were not going as well as they had hoped. Part of the problem is that Vegas is also the center for national and global conferences, conventions, and shows. Many of the potential hydroponic customers can deal wholesale with the manufacturers themselves at these yearly meetings.

Aquaponics (www.buynevada.org/businesses/growers/pur -produce/), where plants grow in water that is nourished by the excretions of fish, or as one specialist informed me "the poo and pee of fish," is also on the rise. With just a little bit of space, a greenhouse, water, some fish, and, oh yes, some know-how, one can grow healthy, tasty produce all year.

An exciting addition to Las Vegas is a new company called Indoor Farms of America (www.indoorfarmsamerica.com). On a recent tour of their indoor aeroponic farm, co-owner Ron Evans gave me an inside look at the amazing produce that can be grown with air, water, and LED lights. Ron was emphatic about the potential for individuals and businesses to take control of their food production. He believes that the "hobby mentality" of urban agriculture can be detrimental to the importance of our food security.

He states that aeroponics is the way to "produce food stocks we can grow ourselves." My mouth began to water at the variety of peppers, arugula, cilantro, and lemon-flavored basil. Go visit Ron and Dave at Indoor Farms of America and check out their Victory Garden specials (www.victoryindoorgardens.com).

You say Garden Tower; I say Tower Garden. It gets a little confusing when it comes to the variety of vertical gardening apparatus. According to Ken McCown, who is heading the research on the feasibility of a food hub in Las Vegas at the College of Design at Iowa State University, many types of technologies are being looked at. For vertical gardening, there are two module types, ZipGrow Towers and the Tower Garden Growing Systems, which are tall and allow for maximum growth in limited space. Another type is my favorite, the Garden Tower, which resembles a large terra cotta flower pot with multiple pockets growing out the sides and a handy composting system right down the middle. All of these technologies have a strong presence in Las Vegas. The representatives from the Garden Tower Project are often at community events and making contributions to school gardens.

An excellent way to virtually visit Vegas before even arriving is to watch some YouTube videos of John Kohler at Growing Your Greens (www.youtube.com/user/growingyourgreens). He has some enthusiastic videos about a variety of alternative home farming options, including aquaponics, composting, and holistic permaculture practices, as well as about visits to the Springs Preserve and many other key garden and agriculture locations.

Green Spaces

Contrary to the fully integrated approach of traditional farms, the urban farms of Southern Nevada take more of a distributed private approach. Many of the farms, garden farms, community gardens, orchards, greenhouses, and community supported agriculture (CSA) programs are concentrating on keeping it local and closing the loop.

For example, when Green Our Planet works with schools to convert water-intensive grass areas to a garden space, the farmers from Garden Farms of Nevada can use the grass removed in composting for other farms.

Produce from weekly farmers' markets are routinely passed out to charitable organizations that find places in need of healthy, free food options.

And while pigs are not on a vegan diet, it is nice to know that RC Farms in Northern Nevada has been feeding their twenty-five hundred pigs the food waste from hotels and casinos. This started fifty years ago and has grown to include twelve hotels providing for one farm.

Las Vegas Community Movers and Shakers

Just like any other city, the majority of the movers and shakers in Las Vegas surrounding the local food movement can be found through social media. There may be more Facebook groups than farms and gardens. There is Seed Library Las Vegas, Las Vegas Clark County, Las Vegas Gardening Club, LV Green Community, Food Hub Strategists for Clark County, GMO-Free Las Vegas, and the list goes on. While many of these are claiming territory for a growing movement, the momentum is undeniable.

Enrique Garcia is a transplant from California. Just like Steve Rypka, he was ready to go back to California. Just a few years ago, there was only one vegan restaurant in town. Enrique says, "The last few years, the vegan movement has exploded."

Advocacy comes in many forms. The Carrot Mob, if you haven't heard of it in your city, supports businesses that are making sustainable changes. The most passive thing is to eat and drink. Before visiting Las Vegas, check out the Carrot Mob site for the next Mob attack, and don't forget your carrot costume (www.youtube.com/watch?v=WY7dvnRCgxI).

Another very active group that is always looking for volunteers to help them serve vegan meals to the homeless is Food Not Bombs (www.foodnotbombslasvegas.org). They serve two weekly potluck-style picnics in Huntridge Circle Park. This food has been collected from farmers' markets and other organizations around town with excess produce.

If you are traveling to Vegas in the fall, Great Basin Permaculture sponsors an all-vegan mesquite pancake breakfast held outdoors in one of the community gardens. Last year it was held at Vegas Roots. This is a fine example of organizations coming together and sharing the benefits of their experiences. For a small fee, you can enjoy homemade vegan pancakes made out of milled flour from the pods of locally harvested mesquite trees. Hot off the grill, you can top your pancakes with melting vegan butter, prickly pear jelly, or pomegranate syrup and enjoy the cool outdoors in a garden setting with other like-minded people. A word of warning, the natural sweetness attracts bees, so leave your bright yellow T-shirt at home.

The pancakes are so delicious that Chef Donald from Vege-Nation has plans to add it to the breakfast menu in an attempt to feature more local fare. VegeNation is also the location for an all-vegan Thanksgiving dinner. VegeNation is so connected with the community that last Thanksgiving they partnered with Green Our Planet to have proceeds sponsor a school garden.

Another inspired, local advocate of sustainable healthy eating is Carlos de Santiago. De Santiago has created an app called *Buymeby*, which allows grocery stores to lower prices of food as it gets closer to the end of its shelf life. This allows users to find food products for a cheaper price and saves food markets massive unsold waste. *Buymeby* has been successfully used in New York, and de Santiago is working hard to bring it to Southern Nevada.

The list of local sustainable food enthusiasts and entrepreneurs continues. For more information, check out the following links. Make your next trip to Vegas a creative, healthy, and enjoyable visit by supporting the movement and its people.

Links
Meet-Ups and Organizations
Angel Face Project
http://projectangelfaces.org/about-us/

Carrot Mob LV
https://www.facebook.com/groups/780177292102439/

Food Hub Strategists for Clark County
https://www.facebook.com/FoodHubClarkCountyNevada/?fref=ts

Food Not Bombs
http://foodnotbombslasvegas.org

Food Not Bombs Las Vegas
https://www.facebook.com/groups/foodnotbombslasvegas

GMO-Free Las Vegas
https://www.facebook.com/GmoFreeLasVegas/?fref=ts

Great Basin Permaculture
http://greatbasinpermaculture.org

Growing Your Greens
https://www.youtube.com/user/growingyourgreens

Las Vegas Clark County Seed Library
https://www.facebook.com/groups/LasVegasClarkCountySeedLibrary

Las Vegas Gardening Club
https://www.facebook.com/groups/521835321215561/

LV Green Community
https://www.facebook.com/groups/268934543230144/

Master Gardeners of Southern Nevada
https://www.facebook.com/MasterGardenersOfSouthernNevada/?fref=ts

Seed Library Las Vegas
https://www.facebook.com/SeedLibraryLasVegas/?fref=ts

Businesses
Garden Farms of Nevada
http://www.gardenfarms.net

Garden Tower Project
http://www.gardentowerproject.com

Indoor Farms of America
http://www.indoorfarmsamerica.com

Urban Hydrogreens
http://www.urbanhydrogreens.com

Wonder Soil
http://wondersoil.com

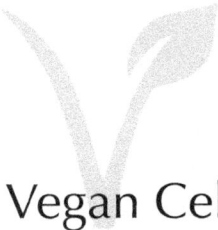

Vegan Celebrities
Marsala Rypka

Hopefully, as human beings, we are always evolving. That has certainly been the case for me in my career, as well as in my food choices.

Like Frank Sinatra, who sang about being a puppet, a pauper, a pirate, a poet, a pawn, and a king, I have had various jobs as a TWA international flight attendant, a Las Vegas talent agent, a nutritional consultant, a celebrity journalist, and most recently a novelist.

With each career change, I learned more about what nourished my heart and soul and what was not satisfying. The same thing pertained to my body. As my consciousness evolved over the years, I went from being a carnivore, to a vegetarian who still consumed dairy products (which are essentially liquid meat), to someone who fully embraces and enjoys a plant-based diet.

I equate the three reasons I gave up the standard American diet (SAD) and became a vegan to a three-legged stool that provides a solid foundation.

The first reason is my health. Fortunately, my husband, Steven, and I found a physician here in Las Vegas, Dr. Evan Allen, who is in alignment with our beliefs and who holds seminars chock-full of scientific evidence that proves fruits, vegetables, grains, and legumes are much healthier than dead animals and their byproducts.

The second reason is because in good conscience I cannot support an industry that raises and slaughters cows, calves, pigs, and chickens in such cruel and inhumane ways just to satisfy humans' lust for flesh. It's hard to stomach, but once you watch *Forks over Knives, Food, Inc., Cowspiracy,* and other food-conscious films, you can never forget the horrors you've seen.

The third reason is because Steven and I care deeply about the future of this wondrous planet with all its natural beauty, and we don't want to continue to contribute to its demise. Mother Earth is in grave danger and it's likely that future generations will not know the world as we do.

Industrial fishing fleets vacuum our oceans until they are devoid of marine life; genetically modified crops (GMOs) contaminate our earth and poison our bodies; and animal livestock produce massive amounts of methane gas, one of the greatest contributors to climate change. All of these things contribute to the collapse of our planet.

Not everyone becomes a vegan for all three of those reasons, but if they do, they are more likely to continue following a plant-based diet because their convictions are deeply rooted in something beyond themselves. If it is just for health reasons, it is easier to fall back into old habits.

As a celebrity journalist for the past twelve years, I have had the opportunity to interview more than one hundred celebrities, including Andre Agassi and Stefanie Graf, Anthony Hopkins, Barry Manilow, Bette Midler, Carlos Santana, Ed Begley Jr., Eva Longoria, Faith Hill and Tim McGraw, Jay Leno, Jerry Rice, Lionel Richie, Mary Steenburgen, Melissa Etheridge, Mick Fleetwood, Olivia Newton-John, Shirley MacLaine, Tony Bennett, Wynonna Judd, and many others.

Someone who may not be as recognizable, but who has a huge presence in Las Vegas and has been very vocal about being vegan, is the iconic casino mogul Steve Wynn. A visionary, Wynn created the momentum that transformed Las Vegas into the sophisticated destination it is today. He imploded landmarks like the Dunes, Desert Inn, and Castaways and replaced them with lavish properties like the Mirage, Treasure Island, and Bellagio (which he later sold to MGM Resorts) and went on to build the magnificent Wynn and Encore resorts.

Steve Wynn helped turn a town known for ninety-nine-cent breakfasts and all-you-can-eat buffets into a world-class city recognized for its celebrity chefs and five-star restaurants. With gourmet eateries like the Wynn's SW Steakhouse and Sinatra at Encore, he wasn't a likely candidate to become a vegan. But then he and his then girlfriend, Andrea Hissom, whom he married in April 2011, had a life-changing experience.

Steve Wynn, Casino Mogul
In June 2010, Wynn and Hissom were vacationing in St. Tropez. They had plans to have dinner with friends—socialite Carol Asher and her multimillionaire boyfriend, Gulu Lalvani. When the two couples got together, Wynn didn't recognize the man Asher was with.

"He looked much younger than Gulu," Wynn told me and the other attendees at a vegan haute cuisine tasting called "Viva Las Vegan," presented by *Bon Appetit* magazine in May 2011 at Encore.

"But it was Gulu. He'd lost about thirty pounds, his eyes were clear, he had a spring in his step, and he looked fifteen years younger. My first thought was that he'd been to a plastic surgeon."

"Gulu, who did you go to?" Wynn asked.

"Nobody," Lalvani replied. "I have a present for you," he said, handing Wynn a DVD titled *Eating*. "Promise me you'll look at it."

That night on their yacht, Wynn and Hissom watched the film. Five minutes into it, Wynn said, "What is this, a diet?" Half-an-hour later, he was not only interested in the health benefits of a plant-based diet, but shocked by the cruelty inflicted upon food production animals. When it was over, the couple decided to go cold turkey and adopt a vegan lifestyle.

The next morning Wynn told the chef on board what they were doing. She immediately got a cookbook out and started preparing great recipes; and they gave all the steaks in the walk-in cooler to their guests.

Once they got back to Las Vegas, Wynn understandably wanted to share this lifestyle change with his employees, since rising health care costs for all of them ran upwards of $60 million a year.

He ordered ten thousand DVDs of *Eating* and distributed them to his employees. He also called Andrew Pascal, then president of Wynn Las Vegas, and said, "I think we should include vegan options in the staff dining room." Pascal went further, posing, "Why don't we give everybody in your hotels a choice?"

For years Wynn was on the drug Lipitor, which kept his cholesterol at 180, but since adopting a plant-based diet, it has reportedly dropped to 140.

"Caring about what you eat and trying to make it tasty and educate the public is not some kind of fringe activity that tree huggers do," says Wynn. "It's a matter of fundamental survival and the continued vitality of our society that starts right here with my family and my employees."

Tal Ronnen, "The Conscious Cook"

In 2010, Steve Wynn enlisted the help of celebrated vegan visionary Tal Ronnen to collaborate with the award-winning chefs at the Wynn and Encore and create an extensive selection of new and innovative vegan options in all the restaurants.

Ronnen, who is known as the "Conscious Cook," a title taken from his 2009 book, *The Conscious Cook: Delicious Meatless Recipes That Will Change the Way You Eat*, became a vegan in 1991.

Since then Ronnen has worked with celebrities like Oprah Winfrey, who, in the spring of 2008, hired him to prepare meals for her twenty-one-day vegan cleanse; Ellen DeGeneres, who hired him to cater her and her partner Portia de Rossi's vegan wedding; and Arianna Huffington, who chose Ronnen as the chef for her party at the Democratic National Convention. He also prepared the first vegan dinner at the U.S. Senate and assisted Chrissie Hynde of the Pretenders in opening the vegan restaurant VegiTerrean in her hometown of Akron, Ohio, which closed in 2011 due to the economic recession.

A graduate of the National Gourmet Institute, Ronnen applies classical French techniques to meatless recipes. Using an array of exotic ingredients and creative preparations, he reinterprets traditional meat-focused dishes into vegan cuisine that tempts and satisfies diners of various tastes.

Ronnen has worked with the chefs at all the fine dining establishments at Steve Wynn's properties, creating vegan appetizer, soup, salad, entrée, and dessert options.

For example, nationally acclaimed chef David Walzog offers hearty dishes such as vegan "clam chowder" with a cashew cream base and smoked oyster mushrooms; Old Bay Cakes with toasted pasta, blistered tomatoes, and ancho-garlic aioli at Lakeside Grill; and Vegan Gardein Beef Skewers with asparagus, sweet peppers, and warm red chili vinaigrette at SW Steakhouse.

Chef Theo Schoenegger, who is at the helm of Wynn's restaurant Sinatra and recently led an interactive cooking class with Ol' Blue Eyes' granddaughter A. J. Lambert, offers decadent dishes such as agnolotti pasta filled with vegan ricotta, herbs, and asparagus sauce.

At Wazuzu, Chef Chen Wei Chan, who was a painter in Taiwan, has artfully added dishes like Gardein Chick'n pot stickers and sweet and sour Gardein Chick'n to the menu.

At Allegro, Chef Enzo Febbraro, who was named Best Chef on the Strip in 2013, includes Gardein Chick'n parmigiano and organic ancient grain penne among his Italian American favorites that retain the authentic flavors of his native Italy.

At Andrea's, the restaurant named in honor of Wynn's wife, Chef Joseph Elevado offers a large selection of vegan Asian-inspired cuisine.

Tal Ronnen offers some wise words when he says, "I hope diners will find that eating meat- and dairy-free cuisine does not have to feel like a sacrifice, but a step up."

Penn Jillette, Entertainer

Magician, juggler, comedian, inventor, and author Penn Jillette, the speaking half of the comedy/magic duo Penn & Teller, which performs at the Rio Hotel and Casino in Las Vegas, recently adopted a vegan diet.

According to publications, including *People* magazine, Penn Jillette, who is 6'7" tall and weighed 330 pounds, suffered from the effects of a poor diet. The entertainer was quoted as saying he felt like crap after every meal, had seasonal allergies and eczema, and would often get sick. At home, he would ration his trips upstairs and pop pain relievers before every show. He said the arthritis in his fingers was getting so bad, he was afraid he'd have to stop doing card tricks. Reportedly, this became the norm for Jillette, who said blood pressure was "a jive-ass thing" and "being fat was no problem."

The wake-up call came when Jillette ended up in the hospital despite the multiple high blood pressure medications he was on. His doctor advised him to have a surgical procedure and get a stomach sleeve. Then the doctor said something that completely blew Jillette's mind. If he could get his weight down to 225 pounds, he probably wouldn't need any of his meds.

In December 2014, Jillette checked with his doctors before embarking on an extremely low one-thousand-calorie diet, which he did until his sixtieth birthday on March 5, 2015.

For two weeks he only ate potatoes. Jillette says he does very well with absolutes. "It's very easy for me to have never had a drink of alcohol in my life, to never have smoked marijuana, but very difficult for me to be a reasonable user. I do better with very hard, fast rules. If I adhere to the rules, my blood pressure goes down."

Jillette continues to follow the advice in Dr. Joel Fuhrman's book *Eat to Live: The Amazing Nutrient-Rich Program for Fast and Sustained Weight Loss.* At 225 pounds, he looks great. He says he did not change his diet for vanity. He was fine with how he looked before. "I liked being a monolith. I happen to like the way I look now more."

Since reaching his goal weight, Penn Jillette has stopped restricting the amounts he eats. "I eat unbelievable amounts of food, just very, very, very healthy food," says the magician.

His typical daily diet consists of an enormous salad with apple cider vinegar as dressing for lunch (he says he doesn't usually eat breakfast). Dinner consists of lots of vegetables and beans with black or brown rice or a vegetable stew, along with lots of fruits for dessert (his favorite is an enormous amount of blueberries with plain cocoa powder), and as a snack, vegetables with vinegar or Tabasco sauce.

Jillette told *People* he could probably have a steak or a dough-nut every couple of weeks, but he just hasn't felt like it. He said when you're feeling as bad as he did, and you start feeling as good as he does, the temptation to go back to doing what you were doing isn't great.

He went on to say that although he didn't exercise during his extreme weight-loss phase, exercise is now fun. Reportedly, he does the "Scientific 7-Minute Workout," along with weight lift-ing, juggling, and ten-mile tricycle rides every other day. Losing the weight has also changed his show. Jillette used to stand. Now he moves around a lot more.

Losing 105 pounds has come with many more pluses than dropping ten pant sizes, like having so much more energy. Jillette says he's just plain happier, something his wife, Emily, and their two children, Moxie CrimeFighter and Zolten, are enjoying.

According to the article, Jillette admits there is one downside. He says he had to get all new suits to wear on stage at the Penn & Teller Show, which he says cost a fortune.

Jillette has said that although he doesn't eat animal products anymore, being called vegan isn't descriptive enough because there are many unhealthy vegans who eat too much processed food.

Though he has insisted he's not a weight-loss messiah, he is quick to admit that he feels better at sixty than he has for the past thirty years.

Mike Tyson, Boxing Heavyweight Champion

In 1982, Bruce Feirstein wrote a tongue-in-cheek book called *Real Men Don't Eat Quiche* that satirized masculine stereotypes. That title became the slogan used by macho-centric men who wanted to justify eating dead animals.

Since then a lot of macho men have debunked that myth, including the former heavyweight boxing champion of the world, Mike Tyson, who adopted a strict vegetarian diet in 2010 and has since lost more than one hundred pounds.

"I was real carnivorous when I was training for fights—I ate lots of meat and cheese. I devoured everything except pork," Tyson told Oprah on her show "Where Are They Now?" He said that as he got older, he didn't like the way he felt. He was so congested from all the drugs and cocaine that he could hardly breathe. He was morbidly obese; had high blood pressure, arthritis, and joint problems; and felt like he was dying.

In 2009, Tyson's four-year-old daughter, Exodus, died in a tragic accident at home, and he told ESPN he didn't want to live anymore.

Then his third wife, Kiki Spicer, watched *Forks over Knives*, and she told her husband she was going to try eating vegan for a month as a way to lose weight.

When Tyson appeared on *The Today Show*, he told Ann Curry that after too many prison cells, too many lawsuits, too many bankruptcies, too many women, too many everything, he knew he had to change his life. What many assumed would be a short-lived experiment soon became a way of life.

"I found out the greatest gladiators in Roman times were vegan," Tyson said. "When scientists did the research they found no meat particles in their bone marrow."

Since then heavyweight boxing champion Mike Tyson has become an unexpected champion of a plant-based diet.

"Becoming a vegan gave me another opportunity to live a healthy life," he says. "I'll always be a fat kid. If I don't watch my diet and exercise and take care myself, my weight balloons up. I was 380; now I weigh 240."

As Tyson told television reporter Greta Van Susteren, "I feel awesome. I wish I was born this way. When I found out about the processed garbage I was eating, it's no wonder I was crazy all those years . . . and the drugs didn't help."

When Tyson tried eating the tiniest piece of meat, he says he got violently sick. "I realized that meat is poison for me now."

Vegan Is Becoming Mainstream

The vegan movement is becoming more mainstream thanks in part to public figures like Al Gore, Alanis Morissette, Alicia Silverstone, Bill Clinton, Casey Affleck, Carrie Underwood, Daryl Hannah, Demi Moore, Ed Begley Jr., Ellen DeGeneres, Ellen Page, James Cameron, James Cromwell, Jason Mraz, Joaquin Phoenix, Kristen Bell, Natalie Portman, Pamela Anderson, Portia de Rossi, Russell Brand, Sandra Oh, Tobey Maguire, Woody Harrelson, and many other celebrities who speak out about the benefits of a plant-based diet.

But we all must take responsibility for spreading the word. Gandhi said, "Be the change you want to see in the world." Hopefully human beings will continue to become more conscious about their health, the well-being of animals, and our long-term survival on the planet.

Professor Mirko Bagaric sums it up when he says: "Suffering is suffering. It is always ugly. It is always unwelcome. It always needs to be stopped. There are no exceptions. A person with the capacity but not the inclination to cease suffering is morally incomplete."

Guidebook to Eating Vegan in Vegas

The Strip

Allegro (The Wynn)

Category:	Vegan-Friendly
Price Range:	$$–$$$
Favorite Eats:	Chick'n Parmigiano
Comments:	Late-night menu.
Contact:	3131 S. Las Vegas Blvd., Las Vegas, NV 89109 (702) 770-2040 www.wynnlasvegas.com
Hours:	5:00 p.m.–6:00 a.m. (Daily) 11:00 a.m.–3:00 p.m. (Lunch)

Andrea's (The Wynn)

Category:	Vegan-Friendly
Price Range:	$$–$$$
Favorite Eats:	Sweet and Sour Gardein Chick'n Vegan Sushi Rolls
Comments:	Asian-inspired cuisine.
Contact:	3131 S. Las Vegas Blvd., Las Vegas, NV 89109 (702) 770-3305 www.wynnlasvegas.com

Hours: Sun–Thurs 6:00 p.m.–10:30 p.m.
                  Fri–Sat 6:00 p.m.–11:30 p.m.

Aureole (Mandalay Bay)

Category: Vegan-Friendly
Price Range: $$$–$$$$
Favorite Eats: Vegan Tasting Menu
Comments: Beautiful restaurant with a large wine tower in the middle. You can order either a vegan tasting plate or the complete tasting menu.
Contact: 3950 S. Las Vegas Blvd., Las Vegas, NV 89119
                  (702) 632-7401
                  www.aurolelv.com
Hours: 5:30 p.m.–10:00 p.m. (Daily)

Border Grill (Mandalay Bay)

Category: Vegan-Friendly
Price Range: $$
Favorite Eats: Crispy California Avocado Tacos
                  Veggie Tacos
Comments: Kitchen is very open to work with you.
Contact: 3950 S. Las Vegas Blvd., Las Vegas, NV 89119
                  (702) 632-7403
                  www.bordergrill.com
Hours: Mon–Thurs 11:00 a.m.–10:00 p.m.
                  Fri 11:00 a.m.–11:00 p.m.
                  Sat 10:00 a.m.–11:00 p.m.
                  Sun 10:00 a.m.–10:00 p.m.

Brio Tuscan Grill (Town Square)

Category:	Vegan-Friendly
Price Range:	$$
Favorite Eats:	Penne Mediterranean (without Cheese)
Comments:	They have a few other menu items that can be modified.
Contact:	6653 S. Las Vegas Blvd., Las Vegas, NV 89119 (702) 914-9145 www.brioitalian.com
Hours:	Sun–Thurs 11:00 a.m.–10:00 p.m. Fri–Sat 11:00 a.m.–11:00 p.m.

The Buffet at the Wynn

Category:	Vegan-Friendly
Price Range:	$$–$$$
Favorite Eats:	Dinner Buffet
Comments:	Vegan entrees and desserts are always available with the greatest selection during the dinner buffet.
Contact:	3131 S. Las Vegas Blvd., Las Vegas, NV 89109 (702) 777-7000 www.wynnlasvegas.com
Hours:	8:00 a.m.–3:00 p.m. (Breakfast; Brunch; Lunch) 3:30 p.m.–10:00 p.m. (Dinner)

Burger Bar (Mandalay Place)

Category:	Vegan-Friendly
Price Range:	$$

Favorite Eats: Vegas Vegan Burger

Comments: Chef Hubert Keller provides a stellar vegan option with veggies between two Portobello mushroom "buns."

Contact: 3930 S. Las Vegas Blvd., Las Vegas, NV 89119
(702) 632-9364
www.burgerbarlv.com

Hours: Sun–Thurs 11:00 a.m.–11:00 p.m.
Fri–Sat 11:00 a.m.–1:00 a.m.

California Pizza Kitchen

Category: Vegan-Friendly

Price Range: $–$$

Favorite Eats: California Veggie Pizza on Thin Crust (No Cheese)
Asparagus and Arugula Salad
Roasted Vegetable Salad
Tomato Basil Spaghettini
White Corn Guacamole and Chips
Dakota Smashed Pea and Barley Soup

Comments: Their corporate website is a model in breaking their menus down for vegetarians, vegans, and those who eat gluten-free. Also located in the Fashion Show Mall.

Contact: 6659 S. Las Vegas Blvd., Las Vegas, NV 89119
(702) 896-5154
www.cpk.com

Hours: Sun–Thurs 11:00 a.m.–10:00 p.m.
Fri–Sat 11:00 a.m.–11:00 p.m.

Costa Di Mare (The Wynn)

Category:	Vegan-Friendly
Price Range:	$$–$$$
Favorite Eats:	Penne al Pomodoro
Comments:	Elegant Italian with some vegan options.
Contact:	3131 S. Las Vegas Blvd., Las Vegas, NV 89109
	(702) 770-3305
	www.wynnlasvegas.com
Hours:	5:30 p.m.–10:00 p.m. (Nightly)

Dal Toro (Inside the Palazzo)

Category:	Vegan-Friendly
Price Range:	$–$$$
Favorite Eats:	Eggplant Carpaccio
	Panzanella Toscana
	Mushroom Risotto
	Avocado Pesto Linguine
	Double Chocolate Brownie
Comments:	Wonderful patio area available. Built around exotic car showroom. Ask hostess for vegan menu before being seated.
Contact:	3325 S. Las Vegas Blvd., Las Vegas, NV 89109
	(702) 437-9800
	www.palazzolasvegas.com
Hours:	7:30 a.m.–11:00 p.m.

Fleur (Mandalay Bay)

Category:	Vegan-Friendly
Price Range:	$$

Favorite Eats: Grilled Vegetable Sandwich
                   Hummus and Baba Ganoush Flatbread Risotto
                   with Scallions (No Cheese)
                   Lemon, Basil, and Pineapple Carpaccio

Comments: Another Hubert Keller restaurant. Better
                   vegetarian selections for dinner than lunch.

Contact: 3950 S. Las Vegas Blvd., Las Vegas, NV 89119
                   (702) 632-9400
                   www.mandalaybay.com/dining

Hours: Sun–Sat 11:00 a.m.–10:30 p.m.

Gilley's (Treasure Island)

Category:	Vegan-Friendly
Price Range:	$$
Favorite Eats:	Gardein BBQ Vegan Chick'n Plate
Comments:	Western restaurant with live music. Most Treasure Island restaurants will have vegan options off the menu.
Contact:	3300 S. Las Vegas Blvd., Las Vegas, NV 89109 (702) 894-7111 www.gilleyslasvegas.com
Hours:	11:00 a.m.–12:00 a.m. (Daily)

Holstein's (Cosmopolitan)

Category:	Vegan-Friendly
Price Range:	$$
Favorite Eats:	Urth Vegan Burger
Comments:	A great vegan burger in the beautiful Cosmopolitan.

Contact:	3708 S. Las Vegas Blvd., Las Vegas, NV 89109 (702) 698-7940 www.holsteinslv.com
Hours:	Sun–Sat 11:00 a.m.–12:00 a.m. Fri, Sat, and Mon 12:00 a.m.–2:00 a.m. (Late Night)

Hussong's Cantina (Mandalay Place)

Category:	Vegan-Friendly
Price Range:	$$
Favorite Eats:	Chick'n Quesadillas Sopes Vegan Street Tacos
Comments:	Hussong's has a full vegan menu. Ask hostess for vegan menu when you come in. Same ownership group as Slice of Vegas Pizza. Now has another location in Summerlin.
Contact:	3930 S. Las Vegas Blvd., Las Vegas, NV 89119 (702) 632-6450 www.hussongslasvegas.com
Hours:	Sun–Thurs 11:00 a.m.–11:00 p.m. Fri–Sat 11:00 a.m.–12:00 a.m.

I Love Burgers (Town Square and Palazzo)

Category:	Vegan-Friendly
Price Range:	$$
Favorite Eats:	Vegan Black Bean Patty (No Bun) I Love Chopped Salad
Comments:	Bun on vegan burger is not vegan, but ordered by itself, it is still very tasty.

Contact:	Palazzo: 3327 S. Las Vegas Blvd., Las Vegas, NV 89109 (702) 242-2747 Town Square: 6605 S. Las Vegas Blvd., Las Vegas, NV 89119 (702) 675-7800 www.iloveburgers.com
Hours:	Mon–Sat 11:00 a.m.–10:00 p.m. (Town Square) Sun–Thurs 8:00 a.m.–11:00 p.m. (Palazzo) Fri–Sat 8:00 a.m.–12:00 a.m. (Palazzo)

Jaleo (Cosmopolitan)

Category:	Vegan-Friendly
Price Range:	$$
Favorite Eats:	Setas al Ajillo con Serena Trigueros con Romesco Escalivada Catalana
Comments:	Top-notch tapas in a beautiful setting.
Contact:	3708 S. Las Vegas Blvd., Las Vegas, NV 89109 (702) 698-7950 www.jaleo.com
Hours:	12:00 p.m.–12:00 a.m. (Daily)

Jardin (The Encore)

Category:	Vegan-Friendly
Price Range:	$$
Favorite Eats:	Vegan French Toast Buffalo Cauliflower
Comments:	Relaxed dining with beautiful views.
Contact:	3131 S. Las Vegas Blvd., Las Vegas, NV 89109

(702) 770-5300
www.wynnlasvegas.com

Hours: Sun–Thurs 7:00 a.m.–11:00 p.m.
Fri–Sat 7:00 a.m.–1:00 a.m.

Julian Serrano (Aria)

Category: Vegan-Friendly
Price Range: $$
Favorite Eats: Padron Peppers
Coca Vegetarian Pizza
Baby Spinach
Comments: Light and airy setting in the Aria in City Center.
Hosts a number of vegetarian items on the menu
that can be modified.
Contact: 3730 S. Las Vegas Blvd., Las Vegas, NV 89158
(877)230-2742
www.arialasvegas.com
Hours: Sun–Thurs 11:30 a.m.–11:00 p.m.
Fri–Sat 11:30 a.m.–11:30 p.m.

Kabuki Japanese Restaurant

Category: Vegan-Friendly
Price Range: $–$$
Favorite Eats: Avocado Roll
Soy Ramen Noodle Bowl
Shishito Peppers
Fried Tofu Avocado Roll
Comments: Also location in Tivoli Village.
Contact: 6605 S. Las Vegas Blvd., Las Vegas, NV 89119

(702) 896-7440
www.kabukirestaurants.com

Hours: Mon–Thurs 11:00 a.m.–10:30 p.m.
               Fri–Sat 11:00 a.m.–11:00 p.m.
               Sun 11:00 a.m.–10:00 p.m.

Lakeside (The Wynn)

Category:	Vegan-Friendly
Price Range:	$$–$$$
Favorite Eats:	Old Bay "Crab Cakes"
	"Clam Chowder"
	Carrot Cake with Pineapple Frosting
	Walnut-Crusted Gardein Chick'n Truffle Arancini
Comments:	An absolutely beautiful restaurant with some of the best vegan meals in Las Vegas.
Contact:	3131 S. Las Vegas Blvd., Las Vegas, NV 89109
	(702) 770-3312
	www.wynnlasvegas.com
Hours:	Sun–Thurs 5:30 p.m.–10:30 p.m.
	Fri–Sat 5:30 p.m.–11:00 p.m.

Le Cave (The Wynn)

Category:	Vegan-Friendly
Price Range:	$$
Favorite Eats:	Roasted Red Pepper, Kalamata Olive, and Marinara Flatbread
	Mushroom Tortellini
Comments:	Romantic restaurant with wine-cave feeling. Great wine selection, patio seating, and late-night lounge on weekends.

Contact:	3131 S. Las Vegas Blvd., Las Vegas, NV 89109 (702) 248-3463 www.wynnlasvegas.com
Hours:	Mon–Thurs 12:00 p.m.–11:00 p.m. Fri–Sun 12:00 p.m.–12:00 a.m.

Mizumi (The Wynn)

Category:	Vegan-Friendly
Price Range:	$$–$$$
Favorite Eats:	Spring Vegetable Roll
Comments:	Another gorgeous Wynn restaurant with one of the best vegan sushi rolls you will find anywhere.
Contact:	3131 S. Las Vegas Blvd., Las Vegas, NV 89109 (702) 770-3320 www.wynnlasvegas.com
Hours:	Sun–Thurs 5:30 p.m.–10:00 p.m. Fri–Sat 5:30 p.m.–10:30 p.m.

Red 8 (The Wynn)

Category:	Vegan-Friendly
Price Range:	$$
Favorite Eats:	Shiitake Tofu
Comments:	Immerse yourself in deep, rich red tones.
Contact:	3131 S. Las Vegas Blvd., Las Vegas, NV 89109 (702) 770-3380 www.wynnlasvegas.com
Hours:	Sun–Thurs 11:00 a.m.–11:00 p.m. Fri–Sat 11:00 a.m.–1:00 a.m.

Ri Ra Irish Pub (Mandalay Place)

Category:	Vegan-Friendly
Price Range:	$–$$
Favorite Eats:	Hummus Pita Sandwich
Comments:	Authentic Irish pub built in Ireland, disassembled, shipped to America, and reassembled in Mandalay Place. Late-night music and fun.
Contact:	3930 S. Las Vegas Blvd., Las Vegas, NV 89119 (702) 632-7771 www.rira.com
Hours:	Mon–Thurs 11:00 a.m.–3:00 a.m. Fri–Sat 11:00 a.m.–4:00 a.m. Sun 11:00 a.m.–3:00 a.m.

Rice and Company (Luxor Atrium at Mandalay Place Entrance)

Category:	Vegan-Friendly
Price Range:	$$
Favorite Eats:	Ma Po Tofu and Stir-Fry Vegetables
Comments:	Trendy Asian
Contact:	3900 S. Las Vegas Blvd., Las Vegas, NV 89119 (702) 262-4852 www.luxor.com
Hours:	Sun–Thurs 5:00 p.m.–10:00 p.m. Fri–Sat 5:00 p.m.–11:00 p.m.

Sinatra (The Encore)

Category:	Vegan-Friendly
Price Range:	$$–$$$

Favorite Eats: Gardein Chick'n Marsala
                   Pennette Pasta with Gardein Sausage

Comments: Upscale Italian dining with lots of memorabilia of
              Ol' Blue Eyes.

Contact: 3131 S. Las Vegas Blvd., Las Vegas, NV 89109
             (702) 770-5320
             www.wynnlasvegas.com

Hours: 5:30 p.m.–10:00 p.m. (Nightly)

Slice of Vegas Pizza (Mandalay Place)

Category: Vegan-Friendly

Price Range: $$

Favorite Eats: Vegan Veggie Pizza
                   Vegan BBQ Chick'n Pizza
                   Vegan Pasta
                   Meatless Meatballs Bruschetta
                   Boneless Chick'n Wings
                   Vegan Garlic Bread
                   Chocolate–Peanut Butter Cake

Comments: Ask hostess for vegan menu as you are seated.

Contact: 3930 S. Las Vegas Blvd., Las Vegas, NV 891119
             (702) 632-6470
             www.sliceofvegaspizza.com

Hours: Sun–Wed 11:00 a.m.–11:00 p.m.
           Thurs–Sat 11:00 a.m.–2:00 a.m.

Sushi Samba (The Palazzo)

Category: Vegan-Friendly

Price Range: $–$$

Favorite Eats: Veggie Kun Roll
Shishito Peppers

Comments: Fun Brazilian, Peruvian, and Asian fusion
restaurant in The Palazzo Shoppes.

Contact: 3327 S. Las Vegas Blvd., Las Vegas, NV 89109
(702) 607-0700
www.sushisamba.com

Hours: Sun–Wed 11:30 a.m.–1:00 a.m.
Thurs–Sat 11:30 a.m.–2:00 a.m.

Tableau (The Wynn)

Category:	Vegan-Friendly
Price Range:	$–$$
Favorite Eats:	Gardein Benedict Blueberry Pancakes
Comments:	Beautiful spot for breakfast or lunch with vegan options.
Contact:	3131 S. Las Vegas Blvd., Las Vegas, NV 89109 (702) 770-3330 www.wynnlasvegas.com
Hours:	7:30 a.m.–11:30 a.m. (Daily; Breakfast) 11:30 a.m.–2:30 p.m. (Daily; Lunch)

Tacos and Tequila (Luxor–Atrium Level)

Category:	Vegan-Friendly
Price Range:	$$
Favorite Eats:	Vegetarian Tacos Salsa and Chips
Comments:	Order the vegetarian tacos without cheese or crema. Outstanding salsa and chips.

Contact:	3900 S. Las Vegas Blvd., Las Vegas, NV 89110
	(702) 262-5225
	www.tacosandtequilalv.com
Hours:	Sun–Sat 11:00 a.m.–11:00 p.m.

Terrace Pointe Café (The Wynn)

Category:	Vegan-Friendly
Price Range:	$$
Favorite Eats:	Baguette French Toast
	Crispy Gardein Chick'n and Waffles
Comments:	Beautiful breakfast and lunch spot with great vegan options.
Contact:	3131 S. Las Vegas Blvd., Las Vegas, NV 89109
	(702) 770-3360
	www.wynnlasvegas.com
Hours:	6:00 a.m.–3:00 p.m. (Daily)

Todd English's P.U.B. (Crystals City Center)

Category:	Vegan-Friendly
Price Range:	$$
Favorite Eats:	Veggie Muffuletta (without Cheese)
Comments:	A must-try sandwich.
Contact:	3720 S. Las Vegas Blvd., Las Vegas, NV 89109
	(702) 489-8080
	www.toddenglish.com
Hours:	11:00 a.m.–12:00 a.m. (Daily)

Tommy Bahama Restaurant (Town Square)

Category:	Vegan-Friendly
Price Range:	$$

Favorite Eats:	Roasted Vegetables with Quinoa
	Spinach and Tomato Pasta (with Olive Oil instead
	of Butter)
Comments:	Restaurant attached to store. Has vegetarian
	menu section with many items that can be
	modified for vegans.
Contact:	6635 S. Las Vegas Blvd., Las Vegas, NV 89119
	(702) 948-8006
	www.tommybahama.com
Hours:	Mon–Thurs 11:00 a.m.–10:00 p.m.
	Fri–Sat 11:00 a.m.–11:00 p.m.
	Sun 11:00 a.m.–9:00 p.m.

Wazuzu (The Encore)

Category:	Vegan-Friendly
Price Range:	$$–$$$
Favorite Eats:	Vegan Drunken Noodles with Crispy Tofu
	Crispy Teriyaki Tofu Bowl
	Vegan Guiltless Brownie
Comments:	Upscale Asian dining with an amazing crystal
	dragon on dining room wall.
Contact:	3131 S. Las Vegas Blvd., Las Vegas, NV 89109
	(702) 770-5388
	www.wynnlasvegas.com
Hours:	Sun–Thurs 11:30 a.m.–10:30 p.m.
	Fri–Sat 11:30 a.m.–1:00 a.m.

Whole Foods Market (Town Square)

Category:	Vegan-Friendly
Price Range:	$–$$

Favorite Eats: Vegan Steam Table Salad Bar
Vegan Pizza
Prepared Foods
Taco Bar Sandwiches
Vegan Burger
Desserts and Baked Goods

Comments: Great place to dine in or take out. Lots of vegan food options for any time of the day. Locations throughout the Valley.

Contact: 6689 Las Vegas Blvd., Las Vegas, NV 89119
(702) 589-7711
www.wholefoodsmarkets.com

Hours: 8:00 a.m.–10:00 p.m. (Daily)

Yard House

Category: Vegan-Friendly

Price Range: $–$$

Favorite Eats: Mediterranean Vegetable Sandwich
Tofu-Mushroom Lettuce Wraps
Gardein Veggie Rice Bowl
Blackened Gardein
Chicken Sandwich Gardein Sliders

Comments: Yard House has a section on their menus featuring Gardein meat and dairy-free products.

Contact: 6593 S. Las Vegas Blvd., Las Vegas, NV 89119
(702) 734-9273
www.yardhouse.com

Hours: Sun–Thurs 11:00 a.m.–1:15 a.m.
Fri–Sat 11:00 a.m.–1:45 a.m.

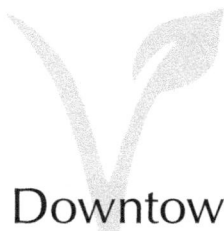

Downtown—Arts District

Arizona Tamale Factory (Downtown 3rd St. Farmers' market)

Category:	Vegan-Friendly
Price Range:	$
Favorite Eats:	Vegan Tamales
Comments:	Arizona Tamale Factory makes about fifteen types of vegan tamales; you can buy one or two hot to eat at the Farmers' Market or take some frozen ones home with you.
Contact:	Stewart and Third St. (Next to Mob Museum in Old Transit Center) www.downtown3rdfarmersmarket.com www.arizonatamalefactory.com
Hours:	Fri 9:00 a.m.–2:00 p.m.

The Beat Coffeehouse

Category:	Vegan-Friendly
Price Range:	$
Favorite Eats:	Roasted Veggie Wrap

Vegetarian Baguette Pizza (No Cheese with
either Hummus or Eggplant Spread)
Quinoa Tabouleh Salad Hummus and Crostini
Plate

Comments: Coffee house in the Emergency Arts Building.
Houses vinyl record shop with vinyl always
playing. A big meeting place in the downtown
area.

Contact: 520 E. Fremont St., Las Vegas, NV 89101
(702) 385-2328
www.thebeatlv.com

Hours: Mon–Fri 7:00 a.m.–12:00 a.m.
Sat 9:00 a.m.–12:00 a.m.
Sun 9:00 a.m.–5:00 p.m.

The Bronze Café (inside the Center)

Category: Vegan-Friendly

Price Range: $–$$

Favorite Eats: Vegucated Sandwich
Guac and Mole Sandwich
The Bizness
Cheezecake

Comments: Wide selection of vegan sandwiches, salads,
pastries, and more. Outstanding food and friendly
service.

Contact: 401 S. Maryland Pkwy., Las Vegas, NV 89101
(702) 202-3100
www.facebook.com/bronzecafelv

Hours: Mon–Fri 10:00 a.m.–10:00 p.m.
Sat 10:00 a.m.–3:00 p.m.

EAT

Category:	Vegan-Friendly
Price Range:	$–$$
Favorite Eats:	Tofu and Mushroom Breakfast Scramble Oatmeal Tofu or Veggie Bánh Mì Sandwich (without Fish Sauce) Vegetarian Chili
Comments:	Chef Natalie has a winner with this hip downtown diner for breakfast and lunch.
Contact:	707 Carson St. (at 7th), Las Vegas, NV 89101 (702) 534-1515 www.eatdtlv.com
Hours:	Mon–Fri 8:00 a.m.–3:00 p.m. Sat–Sun 8:00 a.m.–2:00 p.m.

GrassRoots Juice Bar

Category:	Vegan
Price Range:	$–$$
Favorite Eats:	Green Juices Bud 'n' Vine Smoothie Thai Ginger Soup
Comments:	Organic, local superfood juices, smoothies, and more. Staff is attentive and knowledgeable.
Contact:	124 S. 6th St., Suite 160, Las Vegas, NV 89101 (702) 550-6444 grassrootslv.com
Hours:	Mon–Sat 7:00 a.m.–4:00 p.m.

La Comida

Category:	Vegan-Friendly
Price Range:	$–$$
Favorite Eats:	Veggie Tacos
	Guacamole
Comments:	Great margaritas too.
Contact:	100 S. 6th St., Las Vegas, NV 89101
	(702) 463-9900
	www.lacomidalv.com
Hours:	Mon–Thurs 11:30 a.m.–11:00 p.m.
	Fri–Sat 11:30 a.m.–2:00 a.m.

Le Thai

Category:	Vegan-Friendly
Price Range:	$–$$
Favorite Eats:	Spicy Eggplant with Rice
	Tofu Massaman Curry
	Garlic Fried Rice
Comments:	Excellent Thai food and a bright spot in the downtown area.
Contact:	523 Fremont St., Las Vegas, NV 89101
	(702) 778-0888
	www.lethaivegas.com
Hours:	Mon–Thurs 11:00 a.m.–11:00 p.m.
	Fri–Sat 11:00 a.m.–2:00 a.m.

Lola's—A Louisiana Kitchen

Category:	Vegan-Friendly
Price Range:	$$

Favorite Eats: Cajun Pasta with Veggies

Comments: Nothing on the menu that is plant-based, but
they will whip up a spicy Cajun pasta dish with
veggies for you and it is worth noting.

Contact: 241 W. Charleston Blvd., Las Vegas, NV 89102
(702) 227-5652
www.lolaslasvegas.com

Hours: Mon–Thurs 11:00 a.m.–9:00 p.m.
Fri 11:00 a.m.–10:00 p.m.
Sat 12:00 p.m.–10:00 p.m.

MTO Café

Category: Vegan-Friendly

Price Range: $–$$

Favorite Eats: Vegan Coconut-Carrot Pancakes
Veggie Wrap
Salads
Fresh Juices

Comments: Fantastic spot across from the new city hall. More
vegan-friendly items on the way. Another location
in downtown Summerlin.

Contact: 500 S. Main St., Las Vegas, NV 89101
(702) 380-8229
www.mtocafe.com

Hours: 8:00 a.m.–2:00 p.m.

Mundo (In Las Vegas Design Center)

Category: Vegan-Friendly

Price Range: $$

Favorite Eats: Sweet Corn Tamale
Vegetarian Tacos
Grilled Vegetable Salad
Vegetable Chile Relleno

Comments: Beautiful Nuevo Latino restaurant in the Las
Vegas Design building in the World Market
Center. They have a vegetarian section on menu
that can be modified. Great salsa and chips.

Contact: 995 S. Grand Central Pkwy., Las Vegas, NV
89106
(702) 270-4400
www.mundolasvegas.com

Hours: Mon–Fri 11:00 a.m.–9:00 p.m.
Sat 5:00 p.m.–9:00 p.m.
Open Sun during Broadway shows at the Smith
Center

Nacho Daddy 2

Category: Vegan-Friendly

Price Range: $

Favorite Eats: Spicy Tofu Burrito
Cajun Tofu Street Tacos

Comments: Fun place with solid vegan menu selections near
Fremont St. Experience.

Contact: 113 N. 4th St., Las Vegas, NV 89101
(702) 778-1800
www.nachodaddy.com

Hours: Mon–Fri 7:00 a.m.–2:00 am.
Sat–Sun 9:00 a.m.–2:00 a.m.

Pizza Rock Las Vegas

Category:	Vegan-Friendly
Price Range:	$–$$
Favorite Eats:	Marinara Pizza with No Cheese, Caramelized Onions, and Arugula
Comments:	Come see the "truck," listen to the rock music, and eat late on weekends.
Contact:	201 N. 3rd St., Las Vegas, NV 89101 (702) 385-0838 www.pizzarocklasvegas.com
Hours:	Sun–Thurs 11:00 a.m.–12:00 a.m. Fri–Sat 11:00 a.m.–4:00 a.m.

Pop Up Pizza (Plaza Hotel)

Category:	Vegan-Friendly
Price Range:	$
Favorite Eats:	Vegan Pizza by the Slice Vegan Soft Serve
Comments:	Downtown in the refurbished Plaza Hotel. You can order a whole pie as well.
Contact:	1 Main St., Las Vegas, NV 89101 (702) 366-0049 www.popuppizzalv.com
Hours:	11:00 a.m.–2:00 a.m. (Daily)

Rika Arepa Express

Category:	Vegan-Friendly
Price Range:	$

Favorite Eats: Vegan Arepa with Black Beans, Avocado, and Sweet Plantains

Comments: Food truck with a terrific vegan option. Downtown Farmers Market on Fridays and at various spots throughout the week.

Contact: (702) 762-6360
www.rikaarepaexpress.com

Simply Pure (Container Park)

Category: Vegan/Raw

Price Range: $–$$

Favorite Eats: Raw Chili Cheese Fries
Nachos
Lasagna

Comments: Chef Stacey Dougan has it going on inside of the terrific Downtown Container Park Downtown. Also offers catering and meal service.

Contact: 707 E. Fremont St., Las Vegas, NV 89101
(702) 810-5641
www.chefstaceydougan.com

Hours: Mon–Thurs 11:00 a.m.–9:00 p.m.
Fri–Sat 11:00 a.m.–10:00 p.m.
Sun 11:00 a.m.–8:00 p.m.

VegeNation

Category: Vegan

Price Range: $–$$

Favorite Eats: Save the Tuna (Vegan Sushi)
Muchas Gracias

Pho
Brownie Sundae
Chick'n and Waffles

Comments: A place vegans love that also wins over omnivores with a wide variety of innovative, delicious plant-based dishes.

Contact: 616 E. Carson Ave., Suite 120, Las Vegas, NV 89101
(702) 366-8515
vegenationlv.com

Hours: Mon–Thurs 8:00 a.m.–9:00 p.m.
Fri–Sat 8:00 a.m.–10:00 p.m.
Sun 8:00 a.m.–9:00 p.m.

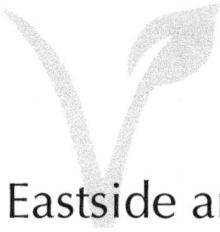

Eastside and Henderson

Bachi Burger

Category:	Vegan-Friendly
Price Range:	$–$$
Favorite Eats:	No Meat Burger (Protein-Style without Bun)
Comments:	Great toppings and makes for a fun and delicious burger even without the bun. Also has a Westside location.
Contact:	470 E. Windmill Ln., Las Vegas, NV 89123 (702) 242-2244 www.bachiburger.com
Hours:	Sun–Mon 12:00 p.m.–11:00 p.m. Tues–Sat 11:00 a.m.–2:00 a.m.

Bangkok 9

Category:	Vegan-Friendly
Price Range:	$–$$
Favorite Eats:	Eggplant Delight
Comments:	Thai and Chinese cuisine with a number of options.

Contact:	663 N. Stephanie St., Henderson, NV 89014
	(702) 898-6881
	www.bangkok9henderson.com
Hours:	11:00 a.m.–10:00 p.m. (Daily)

Bistro Pizza

Category:	Vegan-Friendly
Price Range:	$–$$
Favorite Eats:	Spinach, Mushroom, and Jalapeno Pizza (without Cheese)
Comments:	Very good pizza. Create your own without cheese and choice of veggie options.
Contact:	55 S. Gibson Rd., Henderson, NV 89012
	(702) 558-7330
	www.bistropizzahenderson.com

Bratalian Neapolitan Cantina

Category:	Vegan-Friendly
Price Range:	$$
Favorite Eats:	Spaghetti Al'Aglio, Olio, and Pepperocino
	Penne D'Arrabiatta
	Orecchiette Pugiliese (without Sausage)
	Sorbet Trio
Comments:	A Carla Pellegrino restaurant and one of the best Italian places in the Las Vegas area.
Contact:	10740 S. Eastern Ave. #155, Henderson, NV 89052
	(702) 454-0104
	www.bratalian.com
Hours:	Mon–Sat 5:00 p.m.–10:30 p.m.

Carlito's Burritos

Category:	Vegan-Friendly
Price Range:	$
Favorite Eats:	Veggie Burrito
Comments:	New Mexico–style burritos, order without cheese. These burritos are a handful.
Contact:	4300 East Sunset Road, Henderson, NV 89014 (702) 547-3592 www.carlitosburritos.com
Hours:	Mon–Fri 7:30 a.m.–9:00 p.m. Sat 9:00 a.m.–9:00 p.m. Sun 9:00 a.m.–7:00 p.m.

Cheesecake Factory

Category:	Vegan-Friendly
Price Range:	$–$$
Favorite Eats:	Skinnylicious Veggie Burger Mushroom Lettuce Wraps Vegan Cobb Salad
Comments:	Multiple locations around the Valley.
Contact:	160 S. Green Valley Pkwy., Henderson, NV 89012 (702) 207-6372 www.thecheesecakefactory.com
Hours:	Mon–Thurs 11:00 a.m.–11:00 p.m. Fri–Sat 11:00 am.–12:00 a.m. Sun 10:00 a.m.–11:00 p.m.

Cornish Pasty Co.

Category: Vegan-Friendly

Price Range: $

Favorite Eats: Your choice of a couple of vegan pasties each day.

Comments: Authentic English pub next to Komol.

Contact: 953 E. Sahara Ave., Las Vegas, NV 89101
(702) 862-4538
www.cornishpastyco.com

Coyotes Mexican Cantina

Category: Vegan-Friendly

Price Range: $

Favorite Eats: Vegetarian Enchiladas and Burritos (no Cheese)

Comments: Vegetarian section on the menu.

Contact: 4350 E. Sunset Rd., Henderson, NV 89014
(702) 458-3739

Hours: 11:00 a.m.–10:00 p.m. (Daily)

The Crazy Pita

Category: Vegan-Friendly

Price Range: $

Favorite Eats: Vegetarian Falafel Plate (Minus Feta)

Comments: Located in the District in Henderson.

Contact: 2225 Village Walk Dr., Henderson, NV 89052
(702) 896-7482
www.crazypita.com

Hours: Mon–Sat 10:30 a.m.–9:30 p.m.
Sun 10:30 a.m.–8:00 p.m.

Dang Dee Thai Cuisine

Category:	Vegan-Friendly
Price Range:	$
Favorite Eats:	Mixed Vegetable Stir-Fry (without Oyster Sauce)
Comments:	A number of veg-friendly dishes.
Contact:	6087 S. Pecos Rd. #102, Las Vegas, NV 89120 (702) 228-1668 www.dangdeethaicuisine.com
Hours:	11:00 a.m.–9:00 p.m. (Daily)

Denny's Restaurant

Category:	Vegan-Friendly
Price Range:	$–$$
Favorite Eats:	Vegan Burger
Comments:	Even Denny's gets into the action with their Vegan Burger. Locations all over the Valley.
Contact:	1201 Warm Springs Rd., Henderson, NV 89014 (702) 454-7818 www.dennys.com
Hours:	Open 24 hours

The Egg Works

Category:	Vegan-Friendly
Price Range:	$–$$
Favorite Eats:	Tofu Veggie Scramble Tofu Veggie Burrito

Comments:	These are off the menu items. Substitute tofu for eggs in the veggie scramble and avocado for cheese. Make sure and ask for a side of tomatillo sauce.
Contact:	2490 E. Sunset Rd., Las Vegas, NV 89120 (702) 873-3447 www.theeggworks.com
Hours:	6:00 a.m.–3:00 p.m. (Daily)

Fat Choy

Category:	Vegan-Friendly
Price Range:	$
Favorite Eats:	Tofu and Mushroom Bao Sesame Noodles
Comments:	Chef Sheridan Su's delightful new restaurant in the Eureka Casino.
Contact:	595 E. Sahara Ave., Las Vegas, NV 89104 (702) 794-3464 www.fatchoylv.com
Hours:	8:00 a.m.–10:00 p.m. (Daily)

Firefly Tapas Kitchen and Bar

Category:	Vegan-Friendly
Price Range:	$–$$
Favorite Eats:	Padron Peppers Warm Spinach Salad (No Cheese) Veggies and Lentils
Contact:	3824 Paradise Rd., Las Vegas, NV 89169 (702) 369-3971 www.fireflylv.com
Hours:	11:30 a.m.–2:00 a.m. (Daily)

Flame Kabob

Category:	Vegan-Friendly
Price Range:	$–$$
Favorite Eats:	Veggie Kabob Plate Falafel Wrap with Tahini
Comments:	Persian cuisine made fresh.
Contact:	4440 S. Maryland Pkwy., Las Vegas, NV 89119 (702) 476-5544 www.flamekabobmenu.com
Hours:	Mon–Sat 10:30 a.m.–10:30 p.m. Sun 12:00 p.m.–9:00 p.m.

Go Raw Café

Category:	Vegan/Raw
Price Range:	$–$$
Favorite Eats:	Mexicali and Mediterranean Raw Pizzas Lasagna Bruschetta
Comments:	The original raw vegan restaurant in Las Vegas, with a Westside location as well. Great food and juice bar and lots of resources on raw eating and living.
Contact:	2381 E. Windmill Ln., Las Vegas, NV 89123 (702) 450-9007 www.gorawcafe.com
Hours:	Mon–Sat 8:00 a.m.–8:00 p.m. Sun 8:00 a.m.–5:00 p.m.

Greens and Proteins Healthy Kitchen and Juice Bar

Category:	Vegan-Friendly
Price Range:	$–$$

Favorite Eats: Vegan Flatbread Pizza Raw Lettuce Wraps
                   Raw Macho Nachos
                   Vegan Burger
                   Mock Lettuce Wraps

Comments: Also has full vegan juice and smoothie bar.

Contact: 8975 Eastern Ave., Las Vegas, NV 89123
                   (702) 541-7800
                   www.greensandproteins.com

Hours: 8:00 a.m.–10:00 p.m. Daily

Hofbrauhaus

Category: Vegan-Friendly

Price Range: $–$$

Favorite Eats: Grilled Vegan Sausages with Curry Sauce

Comments: Authentic German beer hall.

Contact: 4510 Paradise Rd., Las Vegas, NV 89169
                   (702) 853-2337
                   www.hofbrauhauslasvegas.com

Hours: Sun–Thurs 11:00 a.m.–10:00 p.m.
                   Fri–Sat 11:00 a.m.–12:00 a.m.

Jason's Deli

Category: Vegan-Friendly

Price Range: $

Favorite Eats: Veggaletta Muffaletta (without Cheese)
                   Veggie Wrapinis
                   Pastas
                   Salads

Comments:	Another Eastside location on Maryland Parkway, one in downtown, and two on the Westside.
Contact:	1281 Warm Springs Rd., Henderson, NV 89014 (702) 898-0474 www.jasonsdeli.com
Hours:	10:00 a.m.–9:00 p.m. (Daily)

Komol Thai Restaurant

Category:	Vegan-Friendly
Price Range:	$
Favorite Eats:	Pad Thai Massaman Curry
Comments:	Plenty of vegan dishes, which are clearly identified. A favorite of local herbivores.
Contact:	953 E. Sahara Ave. #E-10, Las Vegas, NV 89104 (702) 731-6542 www.komolrestaurant.com
Hours:	Mon–Sat 11:00 a.m.–10:00 p.m. Sun 12:00 p.m.–10:00 p.m.

Lemongrass Café

Category:	Vegan-Friendly
Price Range:	$
Favorite Eats:	Pho Coy Dau Hu (Vegan Pho)
Comments:	One of the few places to find a really good vegan pho in town.
Contact:	8820 S. Eastern Ave., Las Vegas, NV 89123 (702) 463-1300 www.yelp.com/biz/lemongrass-café-las-vegas-2

Hours: Mon–Thurs 10:00 a.m.–9:30 p.m.
Fri–Sat 10:00 a.m.–10:00 p.m.
Sun 11:00 a.m.–9:00 p.m.

LYFE Kitchen

Category: Vegan-Friendly

Price Range: $–$$

Favorite Eats: Morning Veggie Wrap
Veggie Burger
Thai Red Curry Bowl

Comments: Chain restaurant with a number of healthy, clearly labeled vegan options.

Contact: 140 S. Green Valley Pkwy. #142, Henderson, NV 89012
(702) 558-0131
www.lyfekitchen.com/locations/nv/henderson

Hours: 8:00 a.m.–9:00 p.m. (Daily)

Merkato Ethiopian Café

Category: Vegan-Friendly

Price Range: $–$$

Favorite Eats: Vegetarian Combo Platter

Comments: Ethiopian food with great flavor and textures enjoyed with authentic injera bread. Wonderful Ethiopian coffee as well.

Contact: 855 E. Twain Ave. #112, Las Vegas, NV 89169
(702) 796-1231
www.ethiopianrestaurant.com/nevada/merkato
.html

Hours: Sun–Sat 11:00 a.m.–1:00 a.m.

Mi Peru

Category:	Vegan-Friendly
Price Range:	$
Favorite Eats:	Aromatic Rice with Vegetables (Ask Them to Make It without Chicken Stock) Fried Corn Cusqueña Beer
Comments:	Peruvian food for something a little different.
Contact:	1450 W. Horizon Ridge Pkwy., Henderson, NV 89012 (702) 220-4652 www.miperugrill.com
Hours:	Sun–Thurs 11:00 a.m.–9:00 p.m. Fri–Sat 11:00 a.m.–10:00 p.m.

Miko's Izakaya

Category:	Vegan-Friendly
Price Range:	$–$$
Favorite Eats:	Hawaiian Roll Popeye the Sailor Roll Veggie Tempura Roll Age Tofu Roll Vegetable Yaki-Soba
Comments:	A popular place for locals and tourists alike. Best selection of vegan sushi in town.
Contact:	500 E. Windmill Ln. #165, Las Vegas, NV 89123 (702) 823-2779 www.mikosushilasvegas.com
Hours:	Tues–Sat 5:00 p.m.–10:30 p.m. Sun–Mon Closed

Mint Indian Bistro

Category:	Vegan-Friendly
Price Range:	$$
Favorite Eats:	Chana Masala
	Chana Chaat
	Dal Tadka
	Desi Salad
	Vegan Roti
	Masala Rice
	Aloo Cauliflower
Comments:	Great vegan options at the lunch buffet.
Contact:	730 E. Flamingo Rd., Las Vegas, NV 89119
	(702) 894-9334
	www.mintbistro.com
Hours:	11:00 a.m.–10:30 p.m. (Daily)

Mothership Coffee Roasters

Category:	Vegan-Friendly
Price Range:	$
Favorite Eats:	Butternut Squash Hand Pie
	Nitro Cold Brew
Comments:	Hip coffee house. Same owners as Sunrise Coffee but a different atmosphere.
Contact:	2708 N. Green Valley Pkwy., Henderson, NV 89014
	(702) 456-1869
	www.mothershipcoffee.com
Hours:	11:00 a.m.–10:30 p.m. (Daily)

Nacho Daddy

Category:	Vegan-Friendly
Price Range:	$–$$
Favorite Eats:	Spicy Tofu Burrito
Comments:	Vegan burrito, nacho, taco, and salad options. Another location in downtown area.
Contact:	9925 S. Eastern Ave., Las Vegas, NV 89183 (702) 462-5000 www.nachodaddy.com
Hours:	Mon–Thurs 11:00 a.m.–10:00 p.m. Fri 11:00 a.m.–11:00 p.m. Sat 9:00 a.m.–11:00 p.m. Sun 9:00 a.m.–10:00 p.m.

Naga Thai Dining

Category:	Vegan-Friendly
Price Range:	$–$$
Favorite Eats:	Evil Jungle Noodles
Comments:	Terrific Thai bistro in Henderson near Black Mountain. Very stylish inside with delectable vegan options clearly marked on the menu.
Contact:	76 W. Horizon Ridge Pkwy., Henderson, NV 89012 (702) 508-2008 www.nagathaidining.com
Hours:	Tues–Sat 11:00 a.m.–10:00 p.m. Sun 11:00 a.m.–9:00 p.m. Mon Closed

Olives Mediterranean Grill

Category:	Vegan-Friendly
Price Range:	$
Favorite Eats:	Whole Wheat Falafel-Stuffed Pita
Comments:	Some more good falafel for the mix.
Contact:	3850 E. Sunset Rd., Las Vegas, NV 89120
	(702) 451-8805
	www.theolivegrill.com

Origin India

Category:	Vegan-Friendly
Price Range:	$$
Favorite Eats:	Baked Eggplant in Hyderabadi Sauce
Comments:	Very appealing Indian restaurant with a number of vegan options. Across from the Hard Rock Hotel and Casino.
Contact:	4480 Paradise Rd., Las Vegas, NV 89169
	(702) 734-6342
	www.originindiarestaurant.com
Hours:	11:30 a.m.–11:30 p.m. (Daily)

The Original Sunrise Café

Category:	Vegan-Friendly
Price Range:	$
Favorite Eats:	Grilled Veggie Wrap
Comments:	Popular local stop for breakfast and lunch.
Contact:	8975 S. Eastern Ave., Las Vegas, NV 89123

(702) 257-8877
www.eatatsunrise.com

Hours: 7:00 a.m.–3:00 p.m. (Daily)

P. F. Chang's

Category: Vegan-Friendly
Price Range: $–$$
Favorite Eats: Buddha's Feast
MaPo Tofu
Coconut Curry Vegetables
Comments: They have a vegetarian section that is mostly vegan.
Contact: 4165 Paradise Rd., Las Vegas, NV 89169
(702) 792-2207
101 S. Green Valley Pkwy., Henderson, NV 89012
(702) 361-5065
www.pfchangs.com

Panera Bread

Category: Vegan-Friendly
Price Range: $
Favorite Eats: Mediterranean Veggie Sandwich (without Cheese)
Comments: Two other Henderson locations and two Las Vegas locations.
Contact: 605 Mall Ring Circle, Henderson, NV 89015
(702) 434-4002
www.panerabread.com
Hours: 6:30 a.m.–9:00 p.m. (Daily)

Panevino Restaurant

Category:	Vegan-Friendly
Price Range:	$$–$$$
Favorite Eats:	Vegan Veggie Burger
	Spinach Tortelloni
	Vegan Risotto
	Mardi Gras Primavera Gnocchi with Vodka Sauce
	Mushroom Meatloaf with Garlic Rosemary Mashed Potatoes
	Chocolate Pudding
	Organic and Vegan Salads
Comments:	Upscale Italian. Full vegan menu with appetizers, entrees, and desserts. A great view of the Strip, sunsets, and the airport. All bread in the restaurant is vegan. Oil-free options available. Let them know you are vegan, and they will take great care of you.
Contact:	246 Via Antonio Ave., Las Vegas, NV 89119
	(702) 222-2400
	www.panevinolasvegas.com
Hours:	Mon–Fri 11:00 a.m.–2:30 p.m. (Lunch)
	Mon–Sat 5:00 p.m.–10:00 p.m. (Dinner)

Parsley Mediterranean Grill

Category:	Vegan-Friendly
Price Range:	$
Favorite Eats:	Falafel Wrap
	Falafel Sandwich
	Falafel Salad
	Hummus Baba Ganoush
	Tabouleh Salad

Comments:	Reasonable prices and everything is super fresh and delicious.
Contact:	6420 S. Pecos Rd., Las Vegas, NV 89120 (702) 489-3189 www.parsleyfmg.com
Hours:	11:00 a.m.–8:00 p.m. (Daily)

Penn's Thai House

Category:	Vegan-Friendly
Price Range:	$
Favorite Eats:	Cashew Nut Veggies
Contact:	724 W. Sunset Rd., Henderson, NV 89011 (702) 564-0162
Hours:	11:00 a.m.–9:00 p.m. (Daily)

Ping Pong Thai

Category:	Vegan-Friendly
Price Range:	$
Favorite Eats:	Swimming Rama with Tofu Red Curry Panang Curry Crispy Garlic Tofu and Veggies Vegetable Spring Rolls Yellow Curry Pad Kee Maw
Comments:	The place is hoppin' at lunch time.
Contact:	2955 E. Sunset Rd., Las Vegas, NV 89120 (702) 228-9988 www.pingpongthailasvegas.com

Hours: Mon–Fri 11:00 a.m.–10:00 p.m.
                 Sat 12:00 p.m.–10:00 p.m.
                 Sun 12:00 p.m.–9:00 p.m.

The Pizza Company

Category: Vegan-Friendly
Price Range: $–$$
Favorite Eats: Vegan Veggie Pizza
                  Calzone
                  Baked Ziti
                  Vegan Burger
Comments: A spot on E. Sunset near Eastern that is a jewel.
                  Some of the best vegan pizza you will find, and
                  they deliver in that area.
Contact: 2275 E. Sunset Rd., Las Vegas, NV 89119
                  (702) 363-9300
                  www.pizzacompanylv.com

Rachel's Kitchen

Category: Vegan-Friendly
Price Range: $–$$
Favorite Eats: Vegetarian Sandwiches and Wraps
                  Oatmeal with Fruit
                  Fresh Juices
Comments: Locations on the Westside, in Summerlin, and in
                  Centennial Hills, as well as downtown.
Contact: 2265 Village Walk Dr., Henderson, NV 89052
                  (702) 522-7887
                  www.rachelskitchen.com

Hours:	Mon–Sat 8:00 a.m.–9:00 p.m.
	Sun 8:00 a.m.–4:00 p.m.

Rainbow's End Café

Category:	Vegetarian and Vegan
Price Range:	$–$$
Favorite Eats:	Vegan Burger
	Raw Romaine Wrap
	Raw Tacos
Comments:	Café located in Rainbow's End Health Food Store, which has been in business since 1977.
Contact:	1100 E. Sahara Ave., Las Vegas, NV 89104
	(702) 737-1338
	www.rainbowsendlv.info
Hours:	Mon–Fri 10:00 a.m.–6:00 p.m. (Café)
	Sat 10:00 p.m.–8:00 p.m.
	Sun 12:00 p.m.–5:00 p.m.

Rika Arepa Express

Contact:	Rika Arepa Express
	(702) 762-6360
	www.rikaarepaexpress.com

Roy's

Category:	Vegan-Friendly
Price Range:	$–$$
Favorite Eats:	Sweet Udon Noodles
	Vegetable Sushi Roll
	Firm Pressed Tofu

Comments:	Ask for vegetarian/vegan menu.
Contact:	620 E. Flamingo Rd., Las Vegas, NV 89119
	(702) 691-2053
	www.roysrestaurant.com
Hours:	Mon–Thurs 5:30 p.m.–9:30 p.m.
	Fri 5:30 p.m.–10:00 p.m.
	Sat 5:00 p.m.–10:00 p.m.
	Sun 5:00 p.m.–9:30 p.m.

Sakun Thai

Category:	Vegan-Friendly
Price Range:	$
Favorite Eats:	Yai Kee Mao
Comments:	Another good choice for Thai food.
Contact:	1725 E. Warm Springs Rd., Las Vegas, NV 89119
	(702) 270-2899
	www.sakunthaionline.com
Hours:	Mon–Sun 11:00 a.m.–10:00 p.m.

Sammy's Woodfired Pizza

Category:	Vegan-Friendly
Price Range:	$$
Favorite Eats:	Vegetarian Pizza
	Sun Dried Tomato, Pine Nuts, and Fresh Basil Pizza
Comments:	Order pizzas on gluten-free crust, with vegan pizza sauce and nondairy cheese for vegan options. They also have some other vegetarian options that can be modified. Four locations on Westside.

Contact:	4300 E. Sunset Rd., Henderson, NV 89014
	(702) 365-7777
	www.sammyspizza.com
Hours:	Sun–Thurs 11:00 a.m.–9:30 p.m.
	Sat–Sun 11:00 a.m.–10:00 p.m.

Settebello

Category:	Vegan-Friendly
Price Range:	$$
Favorite Eats:	Artisan pizzas with lots of topping choices. Order without cheese.
Comments:	Maybe the best crust and sauce ever.
Contact:	140 Green Valley Pkwy., Henderson, NV 89012
	(702) 222-3556
	www.settebello.net
Hours:	11:00 a.m.–10:00 p.m. (Daily)

Shabu-Shabu

Category:	Vegan-Friendly
Price Range:	$–$$
Favorite Eats:	Tofu and Veggie Shabu
Comments:	Cook on your own table in front of you. It is an unusual and fun experience.
Contact:	1263 E. Silverado Ranch Blvd., Las Vegas, NV 89183
	(702) 385-4567
	www.goodstuffusa.com
Hours:	Mon–Fri 12:00 p.m.–3:00 p.m. (Lunch)
	Mon–Fri 5:00 p.m.–9:30 p.m. (Dinner)
	Sat–Sun 3:00 p.m.–9:30 p.m. (Dinner)

Shoku Ramen-Ya

Category:	Vegan-Friendly
Price Range:	$
Favorite Eats:	Spicy Miso Bowl
Comments:	They have vegetarian/vegan options. Be sure to ask for veggie broth and nonegg noodles.
Contact:	470 E. Windmill Ln., Suite 110, Las Vegas, NV 89123 (702) 897-0978 www.facebook.com/ShokuRamen
Hours:	11:00 a.m.–11:00 p.m. (Daily)

Siri Thai

Category:	Vegan-Friendly
Price Range:	$
Favorite Eats:	Pad Kee Mou with Tofu
Comments:	You can never have enough good Thai food.
Contact:	2605 Windmill Pkwy., Henderson, NV 89074 (702) 897-1114 www.sirithailv.com
Hours:	Mon–Thurs 11:00 a.m.–9:30 p.m. Fri–Sat 11:00 a.m.–10:00 p.m. Sun 1:00 p.m.–9:00 p.m.

Stephano's Greek and Mediterranean Grill

Category:	Vegan-Friendly
Price Range:	$
Favorite Eats:	Falafel Breakfast Sliders

Comments: Also a new location in Henderson near Anthem.

Contact: 4632 S. Maryland Pkwy., Las Vegas, NV 89119
(702) 795-8444
www.stephanoslv.com

Hours: Mon–Fri 10:30 a.m.–7:00 p.m.
Sat 11:00 a.m.–7:00 p.m.
Sun Closed

Stick E Rice Thai Café

Category: Vegan-Friendly

Price Range: $

Favorite Eats: Mixed Vegetables with Tofu

Comments: A number of veg-friendly items with a variety of Asian influences.

Contact: 2544 E. Desert Inn Rd., Las Vegas, NV 89121
(702) 696-9700
www.stickerice.com

Hours: 11:00 a.m.–9:30 p.m.

Sunrise Coffee

Category: Vegan-Friendly

Price Range: $

Favorite Eats: Alien Burrito Tofurky Sandwich
Nom Nom Burrito
Morning Crunches
Chili Burrito
Vegan Pastries

Comments: A great staff and atmosphere with vegan baked goods by Danielle Russo's Sweet Tooth Bakery.

Contact:	3130 E. Sunset Rd., Las Vegas, NV 89120
	(702) 433-3304
	www.sunrisecoffeelv.com
Hours:	Mon–Fri 6:00 a.m.–8:00 p.m.
	Sat 7:00 a.m.–8:00 p.m.
	Sun 7:00 a.m.–6:00 p.m.

Sweet Tooth Bakery

Category:	Vegan
Price Range:	$
Favorite Eats:	Vegan Muffins
	Vegan Cakes
	Vegan Cookies
Comments:	You can find products at Sunrise Coffee or by special order.
Contact:	(702) 494-8486
	sweettoothvegas@gmail.com
	www.facebook.com/pages/Sweet-Tooth -VeganVegetarian-Bakery

Table Thai

Category:	Vegan-Friendly
Price Range:	$–$$
Favorite Eats:	Vegan Pizzas
	Vegan Soups
	Vegan Salads
	Vegan Sandwiches
	Vegan Desserts

Comments:	Vegan menu. Dine in or take out (order online option). Delivery in the area.
Contact:	3130 E. Sunset Rd., Las Vegas, NV 89120 (702) 779-9366 tablethailasvegas.com

Taco Y Taco

Category:	Vegan-Friendly
Price Range:	$
Favorite Eats:	Burrito with Soyrizo Tacos Burritos Bowls
Comments:	Popular Eastside location now with new location on Eastern.
Contact:	3430 E. Tropicana Ave., Las Vegas, NV 89121 (702) 331-3015 www.tacotacolv.com

Thai Chili

Category:	Vegan-Friendly
Price Range:	$
Favorite Eats:	Pineapple/Veggie Curry
Comments:	Thai Chili has a number of vegan-friendly items.
Contact:	2879 N. Green Valley Pkwy., Henderson, NV 89014 (702) 454-7606 www.facebook.com/pages/Thai-Chili
Hours:	11:00 a.m.–9:00 p.m. (Daily)

Tiabi Coffee and Waffle Bar

Category:	Vegan-Friendly
Price Range:	$
Favorite Eats:	Vegan Waffles
	Churro Waffle with Ice Cream
	Vegan Guru Burger
	Smoothies
Comments:	Delicious waffles and almost everything you can do with waffles.
Contact:	3961 Maryland Pkwy., Las Vegas, NV 89103
	(702) 222-1722
	www.iwanttiabi.com

Whole Foods Market

Category:	Vegan-Friendly
Price Range:	$–$$
Favorite Eats:	Hot Vegan Buffet
	Salad Bar
	Deli Case
	Vegan Pizza
Comments:	Always great vegan options at Whole Foods Market.
Contact:	100 S. Green Valley Pkwy., Henderson, NV 89012
	(702) 361-8183
	6689 Las Vegas Blvd., Las Vegas, NV 89119
	(702) 589-7711
	www.wholefoodsmarket.com
Hours:	8:00 a.m.–10:00 p.m. (Daily)

Winchell's Pub and Grill

Category:	Vegan-Friendly
Price Range:	$–$$
Favorite Eats:	Veggie Pita (without Cheese)
Comments:	Nice little neighborhood pub and a great place to watch a game.
Contact:	199 E. Warm Springs Rd., Las Vegas, NV 89119 (702) 309-7600 www.winchellspub.com
Hours:	Open 24 hours

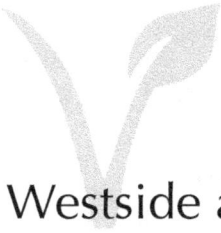

Westside and Northwest

Abyssinia Ethiopian Restaurant

Category:	Vegan-Friendly
Price Range:	$–$$
Favorite Eats:	Vegetarian/Vegan Platter
Comments:	Spicy mounds of delight to scoop up with injera bread.
Contact:	4780 W. Tropicana Ave. #108, Las Vegas, NV 89103 (702) 220-5304 www.ethiopianrestaurant.com/missouri/abyssinia.html
Hours:	Mon–Sun 11:00 a.m.–2:00 a.m.

Aranya Thai Bistro

Category:	Vegan-Friendly
Price Range:	$
Favorite Eats:	Pad Krapow with Tofu and Brown Rice
Comments:	Another solid Thai offering on the Westside of town.

Contact:	4195 S. Grand Canyon Dr., Las Vegas, NV 89147 (702) 243-1912 www.aranyathaibistro.com
Hours:	Mon–Thurs 11:00 a.m.–9:30 p.m. Fri–Sat 11:00 a.m.–10:00 p.m. Sun 3:00 p.m.–9:00 p.m.

Bachi Burger

Category:	Vegan-Friendly
Price Range:	$–$$
Favorite Eats:	No Meat Burger (Protein-Style without Bun)
Comments:	Also has Eastside location.
Contact:	9410 W. Sahara Ave., Las Vegas, NV 89117 (702) 255-3055 www.bachiburger.com
Hours:	Sun–Mon 12:00 p.m.–11:00 p.m. Tues–Sat 11:00 a.m.–12:00 a.m.

The Baguette Café

Category:	Vegan-Friendly
Price Range:	$
Favorite Eats:	Tomato Basil Soup Vegan Panini Veggie Wrap Eggplant Sandwich
Comments:	Very vegan-friendly. Artistic and delicious food.
Contact:	8359 W. Sunset Rd., Las Vegas, NV 89113 (702) 269-4781 www.facebook.com/pages/Baguette-Cafe

Hours:	Mon–Fri 7:00 a.m.–5:00 p.m.
	Sat–Sun Closed

Basil 'n Lime

Category:	Vegan-Friendly
Price Range:	$$
Favorite Eats:	Pad See Ew with Tofu (instead of Meat and Eggs)
Comments:	Good Thai food with some plant-based options.
Contact:	3665 S. Ft. Apache Rd., Las Vegas, NV 89147 (702) 255-2581

Bite Vegan Bakery

Category:	Vegan
Price Range:	$
Favorite Eats:	Raspberry-Chocolate Cake Peanut Butter–Chocolate Chip Mini Cookies
Comments:	Find them at the fresh52 Farmers' Market on Saturdays at Tivoli Village or via special orders.
Contact:	www.ivebeenbitten.com holly@ivebeenbittten.com
Hours:	Saturdays 8:00 a.m.–1:00 p.m. (At fresh52 Farmers' Market in Tivoli Village)

Blaze Pizza

Category:	Vegan-Friendly
Price Range:	$
Favorite Eats:	Veg Out Pizza

Comments: Offers vegan cheese. Also has a Henderson
               location.

Contact: 6211 N. Decatur Blvd., Las Vegas, NV 89130
               (702) 685-47709
               www.blazepizza.com

Hours: 11:00 a.m.–10:00 p.m. (Daily)

Blue Nile Ethiopian

Category: Vegan-Friendly

Price Range: $

Favorite Eats: Vegetarian Platter

Comments: Book a coffee ritual if you can.

Contact: 4180 W. Desert Inn Rd., Las Vegas, NV 89102
                (702) 485-4158

CheeBurger CheeBurger

Category: Vegan-Friendly

Price Range: $

Favorite Eats: Portobello Mushroom Burger

Comments: They are willing work with you to make it work
                for you. Ask them to leave the cheese off the
                burger. The caramelized onions are great.

Contact: 8390 S. Rainbow Blvd., Las Vegas, NV 89139
                (702) 220-3912
                www.cheeburger.com

Hours: Sun–Thurs 11:00 a.m.–9:00 p.m.
                Fri–Sat 11:00 a.m.–10:00 p.m.

Chipotle

Category:	Vegan-Friendly
Price Range:	$
Favorite Eats:	Vegetarian Bowl or Burrito
Comments:	Fresh and delicious with many locations in the Las Vegas and Henderson area.
Contact:	9240 W. Sahara Ave., Las Vegas, NV 89117 (702) 243-0226 www.chipotle.com
Hours:	11:00 a.m.–10:00 p.m. (Daily)

The Daily Kitchen and Wellness Bar

Category:	Vegan-Friendly
Price Range:	$–$$
Favorite Eats:	Pasta Primavera Tuscan Kale Salad
Comments:	Some good plant-based options and a fresh juice bar.
Contact:	3645 S. Town Center Dr., Las Vegas, NV 89135 (702) 685-7100 www.dkeatery.com
Hours:	Mon–Sat 7:00 a.m.–7:00 p.m. Sun 7:00 a.m.–4:00 p.m.

Dom DeMarco's Pizzeria

Category:	Vegan-Friendly
Price Range:	$–$$
Favorite Eats:	Bella Napoli Pizza

Comments:	Has some other plant-based options. Offers nondairy cheese to add to any pizza and a gluten-free crust option.
Contact:	9785 Charleston Blvd., Las Vegas, NV 89117 (702) 570-7000 www.domdemarcos.com
Hours:	Sun–Thurs 11:30 a.m.–9:00 p.m. Fri–Sat 11:30 a.m.–10:00 p.m.

Due Forni

Category:	Vegan-Friendly
Price Range:	$$
Favorite Eats:	Margherita Pizza (No Cheese) with Mushrooms and Caramelized Onions
Comments:	Great pizza made blisteringly fast in one of their nine-hundred-degree ovens.
Contact:	3555 S. Town Center Dr., Las Vegas, NV 89135 (702) 586-6500 www.dueforni.com
Hours:	Sun–Thurs 11:00 a.m.–10:00 p.m. Fri–Sat 11:00 a.m.–11:00 p.m.

DW Bistro

Category:	Vegan-Friendly
Price Range:	$$
Favorite Eats:	DW Veggie Burger with Sweet Potato Fries Veggie Curry Bowl
Comments:	Delicious options here.
Contact:	6115 S. Ft. Apache Rd., Las Vegas, NV 89148

(702) 527-5200

www.dwbistro.com

Hours: Tues–Thurs 11:00 a.m.–3:00 p.m.,
5:00 p.m.–9:00 p.m.
Fri 11:00 a.m.–11:00 p.m.
Sat 10:00 a.m.–11:00 p.m.
Sun 10:00 a.m.–2:00 p.m.

Elevated Juice

Category:	Vegan-Friendly
Price Range:	$–$$
Favorite Eats:	Acai Bowls
	Coffee and Espresso Drinks
	Green Juices
Comments:	Offers juice cleanse packages.
Contact:	7703 N. El Capitan Way, Suite 140, Las Vegas, NV 89143
	(702) 305-2463
	www.drinkelevatedjuice.com
Hours:	Mon–Fri 7:00 a.m.–7:00 p.m.
	Sat–Sun 8:00 a.m.–7:00 p.m.

Go Raw Café

Category:	Vegan/Raw
Price Range:	$–$$
Favorite Eats:	Mexicali Pizza
	Mediterranean Pizza
	Coconut-Curry Vegetables
	Italian Sampler Plate

Comments:	Great food and resources for a raw vegan lifestyle. Another location in Henderson.
Contact:	2910 Lake East Dr., Las Vegas, NV 89117 (702) 254-5382 www.gorawcafe.com
Hours:	Mon–Sat 9:00 a.m.–9:00 p.m. Sun 9:00 a.m.–5:00 p.m.

Go Vegan Café

Category:	Vegetarian and Vegan/Raw
Price Range:	$
Favorite Eats:	Pancakes Waffles Tofu Scrambles Lentil Loaf Cheese Fries
Comments:	Same owners as Go Raw Café. Serves raw and cooked food. Salad bar and juice bar. Breakfast served all day.
Contact:	5875 S. Rainbow Blvd., Las Vegas, NV 89118 (702) 405-8550 www.govegan.cafe
Hours:	Mon–Sat 9:00 a.m.–8:00 p.m. Sun 9:00 a.m.–5:00 p.m.

Greens and Proteins

Category:	Vegan-Friendly
Price Range:	$–$$
Favorite Eats:	Tofu Fries

Thai Ginger Soup

Build Your Own Custom Meal

Comments: Sandwiches, salads, wraps, pizza, smoothies, juices, and more. Also two Eastside locations.

Contact: 6180 N. Decatur Blvd., Las Vegas, NV 89130
(702) 853-0650
6375 S. Rainbow Blvd., Las Vegas, NV 89118
(702) 823-4600
www.greensandproteins.com

Hours: Mon–Sun 7:00 a.m.–10:00 p.m.

Hash House a Go Go

Category: Vegan-Friendly

Price Range: $–$$

Favorite Eats: Portobello Burger (with No Cheese, Add Some Spinach Instead)

Comments: Restaurants with legendary big portions. Not many plant-based options, but the Portobello Burger is good. Also has locations in the M Resort, Plaza Hotel (downtown), and the Quad (on the Strip).

Contact: 6800 W. Sahara Ave., Las Vegas, NV 89146
(702) 804-4646
www.hashhouseagogo.com

Hours: Sun–Thurs 7:30 a.m.–2:30 p.m.,
5:00 p.m.–9:00 p.m.
Fri–Sat 7:30 a.m.–2:30 p.m.,
5:00 p.m.–10:00 p.m.

Jacques Café

Category:	Vegan-Friendly
Price Range:	$–$$
Favorite Eats:	Veggie Burger
	Quinoa Plate
Comments:	Casual American bistro in Summerlin with healthy vegan options.
Contact:	1910 Village Center Drive, Unit 1, Las Vegas, NV 89134
	(702) 550-6363
	www.jacquescafe.vegas
Hours:	Mon–Sat 9:00 a.m.–9:00 p.m.
	Sun 8:00 a.m.–2:00 p.m.

Kabuki Japanese Restaurant

Category:	Vegan-Friendly
Price Range:	$–$$
Favorite Eats:	Spicy Tofu on Crispy Rice
	Shitake Tofu
	Veggie Wrap Combo
	Rainbow Roll
	Ramen Bowl
Comments:	Located in Tivoli Village. Also has a location in Town Square.
Contact:	400 S. Rampart Blvd., Las Vegas, NV 89145
	(702) 685-8877
	www.kabukirestaurants.com

The King and I Thai

Category:	Vegan-Friendly
Price Range:	$
Favorite Eats:	Vegetable Curry
Comments:	In the Lakes in the same shopping center as Go Raw Café.
Contact:	2904 Lake East Dr., Las Vegas, NV 89117
	(702) 256-1568
	www.thairestaurantkingandIatthelakes.com
Hours:	Mon–Thurs 11:00 a.m.–9:30 p.m.
	Fri–Sat 11:00 a.m.–10:00 p.m.
	Sun 3:00 p.m.–9:00 p.m.

Komex Fusion Express

Category:	Vegan-Friendly
Price Range:	$
Favorite Eats:	Fusion Taco
	Fusion Burrito
Comments:	Korean-Mexican fusion. This place rocks it!
Contact:	633 N. Decatur Blvd., Las Vegas, NV 89107
	(702) 646-1612
	4155 S. Buffalo Dr., Las Vegas, NV 89147
	(702) 778-5566
	www.komexexpress.com
Hours:	Mon–Sat 11:00 a.m.–8:00 p.m.
	Sun Closed

Kona Grill

Category:	Vegan-Friendly
Price Range:	$–$$

Favorite Eats: Spicy Garlic Edamame
                   Vegetarian Roll
                   Spicy Udon Noodles

Comments: Ask for vegan menu.

Contact: 750 S. Rampart Blvd., Las Vegas, NV 89145
                   (702) 547-5542
                   www.konagrill.com

Hours: Mon–Thurs 11:00 a.m.–11:00 p.m.
                   Fri–Sat 11:00 a.m.–12:00 a.m.
                   Sun 11:00 a.m.–10:00 p.m.

Kyara Japanese Tapas

Category:	Vegan-Friendly
Price Range:	$–$$
Favorite Eats:	Tofu Steak
	Healthy Kushi Mari
Comments:	Inventive Japanese small plates. Popular late-night hangout for foodies.
Contact:	6555 S. Jones Blvd. #120, Las Vegas, NV 89118
	(702) 434-8856
	www.facebook.com/kyaralv
Hours:	Mon–Sun 11:00 a.m.–3:00 p.m. (Lunch)
	Mon–Sun 5:00 p.m.–2:00 a.m. (Dinner)

Lee's Sandwiches

Category:	Vegan-Friendly
Price Range:	$
Favorite Eats:	Vegetarian Sandwich
Comments:	One of the better sandwich deals in town. Second location in Henderson.

Contact:	3989 Spring Mountain Rd., Las Vegas, NV 89102 (702) 331-9999 www.leessandwiches.com
Hours:	Open 24 hours

MacShack

Category:	Vegan-Friendly
Price Range:	$–$$
Favorite Eats:	Veggie Bowl
Comments:	Sister restaurant to Nora's. Load up the pasta with all the veggies you want. Topped with baked bread crumbs.
Contact:	8680 W. Warm Springs Rd., Las Vegas, NV 89148 (702) 463-2433 8975 W. Charleston Blvd., Las Vegas, NV 89117 (702) 243-1722 www.macaronishack.com
Hours:	Sun–Thurs 11:00 a.m.–9:00 p.m. Fri–Sat 11:00 a.m.–10:00 p.m.

Makino

Category:	Vegan-Friendly
Price Range:	$$
Favorite Eats:	Cucumber Rolls Vegetable Rolls Avocado Rolls Salad Bar

Comments: Japanese buffet with some vegan-friendly options.
                   Also has a location in the Las Vegas Premium
                   Outlets North.

Contact: 3965 S. Decatur Blvd., Las Vegas, NV 89103
                   (702) 884-4477
                   www.makinobuffet.com

Hours: Mon–Thurs 11:30 p.m.–2:30 p.m.,
                   5:30 p.m.–9:00 p.m.
                   Fri–Sun 11:30 p.m.–3:00 p.m.,
                   5:30 p.m.–9:00 p.m.

Mt. Everest India's Cuisine

Category: Vegan-Friendly

Price Range: $–$$

Favorite Eats: Chana Masala

Comments: A handful of vegan options available.

Contact: 3461 W. Sahara Ave., Las Vegas, NV 89102
                   (702) 892-0950
                   www.everestcuisine.net

Hours: 11:00 a.m.–3:00 p.m., 5:00–10:30 p.m. (Daily)

Nora's Cuisine

Category: Vegan-Friendly

Price Range: $$

Favorite Eats: Pasta Primavera
                   Veggie Pizza (No Cheese)

Comments: Terrific Italian food.

Contact: 6020 W. Flamingo Rd., Las Vegas, NV 89103
                   (702) 873-8990
                   www.norascuisine.com

Hours: Mon–Thurs 11:00 a.m.–10:00 p.m.
Fri 11:00 a.m.–12:00 a.m.
Sat 4:00 p.m.–12:00 a.m.
Sun 4:00 p.m.–9:00 p.m.

P. F. Chang's

Category: Vegan-Friendly

Price Range: $–$$

Favorite Eats: Buddha's Feast
MaPo Tofu
Coconut Curry Vegetables

Comments: Two other Las Vegas locations and one Henderson location.

Contact: 1095 S. Rampart Blvd., Las Vegas, NV 89145
(702) 968-8885
www.pfchangs.com

Hours: Mon–Fri 11:00 a.m.–10:00 p.m.

Pan Asian

Category: Vegan-Friendly

Price Range: $–$$

Favorite Eats: Garlic Pepper Sauce and Veggie Stir-Fry

Comments: Great food with some solid plant-based options.

Contact: 2980 S. Durango Dr., Las Vegas, NV 89117
(702) 629-7464
www.davidwongspanasian.com

Hours: Mon–Sat 11:00 a.m.–9:30 p.m.
Sun 11:00 a.m.–9:00 p.m.

Pancho's Kitchen

Category:	Vegan-Friendly
Price Range:	$
Favorite Eats:	Potato Tacos
	Fried Avocado Tacos
	Tamales
Comments:	Authentic Mexican food. Ask for vegan menu.
	Also sold at farmers' markets around town.
Contact:	3655 S. Durango Dr., Suite 27, Las Vegas, NV 89147
	(702) 370-0987
	www.facebook.com/panchoskitchenlv/
Hours:	Mon 10:00 a.m.–6:00 p.m.
	Tues–Fri 10:00 a.m.–8:00 p.m.
	Sat 10:00 a.m.–6:00 p.m.

The Perfect Scoop

Category:	Vegan-Friendly
Price Range:	$
Favorite Eats:	Vegan Brownie Sundae
Comments:	Delicious vegan ice cream in flavors like vanilla,
	cookies 'n' cream, mango, lychee, pineapple,
	green tea, and avocado.
Contact:	5035 S. Ft. Apache Rd., Las Vegas, NV 89148
	(702) 701-7888
	7377 S. Jones Blvd, Las Vegas, NV 89139
	4568 Spring Mountain Rd., Las Vegas, NV 89102
	www.perfectscooplv.com
Hours:	11:30 a.m.–10:00 p.m. (Daily)

Qdoba Mexican Grill

Category:	Vegan-Friendly
Price Range:	$
Favorite Eats:	Vegetarian Burrito
Comments:	Also has a location on Stephanie Rd. in Henderson.
Contact:	5045 W. Tropicana Rd., Las Vegas, NV 89103 (888)587-3622 www.qdoba.com

Rachel's Kitchen

Category:	Vegan-Friendly
Price Range:	$–$$
Favorite Eats:	Vegetarian Sandwiches and Wraps Oatmeal with Fruit Fresh Juices
Comments:	They have a number of vegetarian items that can be modified to be vegan. Has locations in downtown (in the Ogden), Summerlin, and Centennial Hills.
Contact:	3330 S. Hualapai Way, Las Vegas, NV 89117 (702) 459-6789 7010 N. Durango Dr. #140, Las Vegas, NV 89149 (702) 802-5000 9691 Trailwood Dr., Las Vegas, NV 89134 (702) 317-7000 www.rachelskitchen.com
Hours:	Mon–Sat 7:00 a.m.–7:00 p.m. Sun 7:00 a.m.–4:00 p.m.

Rani's World Market and Kitchen

Category:	Vegan-Friendly
Price Range:	$
Favorite Eats:	Indian Sampler Plate
Comments:	Great Indian market and café.
Contact:	4505 W. Sahara Ave., Las Vegas, NV 89102 (702) 522-7744 www.ranisworldfoods.com
Hours:	10:00 a.m.–9:00 p.m. (Daily)

Red Velvet Café

Category:	Vegan-Friendly
Price Range:	$–$$
Favorite Eats:	Veggie Grill Panini Red Velvet Cake Vegan Taco Salad Chocolate Chip Cookies Buffalo Chick'n Panini Teriyaki Mushroom Chick'n Sandwich
Comments:	Almost everything on the menu can be prepared vegan. Nearly all the desserts are vegan and are incredible. All vegan food is prepared in a separate work station in the kitchen.
Contact:	7875 W. Sahara Ave., Las Vegas, NV 89117 (702) 360-1972 www.redvelvetcafelv.com
Hours:	9:00 a.m.–9:00 p.m. (Daily)

Ronald's Donuts

Category:	Vegan-Friendly
Price Range:	$
Favorite Eats:	Vegan Apple Fritters Soy Cream-Filled
Comments:	Vegan donuts? Oh yeah. Ask which donuts are vegan—usually the top two rows. Cash only. These are what legends are made of.
Contact:	4600 Spring Mountain Rd., Las Vegas, NV 89102 (702) 873-1032
Hours:	Mon–Sat 4:00 a.m.–4:00 p.m. Sun 4:00 a.m.–2:00 p.m.

Rubio's

Category:	Vegan-Friendly
Price Range:	$
Favorite Eats:	Healthy Veggie Mex Burrito Grilled Portobello and Poblano Tacos
Comments:	Great fast-food options with delicious plant-based possibilities. Has locations all over the Las Vegas Valley.
Contact:	9310 W. Sahara Ave., Las Vegas, NV 89117 (702) 804-5860 www.rubios.com
Hours:	Mon–Thurs 10:00 a.m.–9:00 p.m. Fri–Sat 10:00 a.m.–9:30 p.m. Sun 11:00 a.m.–9:00 p.m.

Saffron Flavors of India

Category:	Vegan-Friendly
Price Range:	$–$$
Favorite Eats:	Vegetable Samosas Chana Masala Aloo Gobi
Comments:	Vegetarian section on the menu. Many items are vegan or can be modified. Servers are helpful and knowledgeable.
Contact:	4450 N. Tenaya Way, Suite 115, Las Vegas, NV 89129 (702) 489-7900 saffronflavorsofindia.com/index.htm
Hours:	Mon Closed Wed–Sat 11:30 a.m.–2:30 p.m. (Lunch Buffet) Tues–Thurs 5:00 p.m.–9:00 p.m. (Dinner) Fri–Sat 5:00 p.m.–10:00 p.m. (Dinner) Sun 5:00 p.m.–9:00 p.m. (Dinner)

Sammy's Woodfired Pizza

Category:	Vegan-Friendly
Price Range:	$–$$
Favorite Eats:	Vegetarian Pizza Sun Dried Tomato Pizza with Pine Nuts and Fresh Basil
Comments:	Make sure the pizza is made with a gluten-free crust, vegan sauce, and nondairy cheese.
Contact:	6500 W. Sahara Ave., Las Vegas, NV 89146 (702) 227-6000

7345 Arroyo Crossing Pkwy., Las Vegas, NV 89113
(702) 263-7171
9516 W. Flamingo Ave., Las Vegas, NV 89147
(702) 638-9500
7160 N. Durango Dr., Las Vegas, NV 89149
(702) 365-7777
www.sammyspizza.com

Skinny Fats

Category:	Vegan-Friendly
Price Range:	$–$$
Favorite Eats:	Chili-Garlic Edamame
	Buddha's Law Salad
Comments:	Could offer more than it does. Near the Strip.
Contact:	6261 Dean Martin Dr., Las Vegas, NV 89118
	(702) 979-9797
	www.skinnyfats.com
Hours:	Mon–Fri 8:00 a.m.–8:00 p.m.

Surang's Thai Kitchen

Category:	Vegan-Friendly
Price Range:	$–$$
Favorite Eats:	Garlic and Pepper Stir Fry with Tofu
Comments:	Another good option along Ft. Apache Rd.
Contact:	5455 S. Ft. Apache Rd., Las Vegas, NV 89148
	(702) 385-0021
	www.surangthaikitchen.com
Hours:	11:00 a.m.–10:00 p.m. (Daily)

Thai-Style Noodle House #2

Category:	Vegan-Friendly
Price Range:	$–$$
Favorite Eats:	Rad-Na
Comments:	Ask for separate vegan menu. Original location in Chinatown.
Contact:	5135 S. Ft. Apache Rd., Las Vegas, NV 89147
	(702) 823-2882
	www.thainoodle.webs.com
	2267 N. Rampart Blvd., Las Vegas, NV 89134
	(702) 749-7991
	7377 S. Jones Blvd. #113–114, Las Vegas, NV 89139
	(702) 534-7799
Hours:	11:00 a.m.–10:00 p.m.

Trader Joe's

Category:	Vegan-Friendly
Favorite Eats:	Packaged Hummus Wrap
	Spicy Lentil Wrap
	Chickenless Wrap
Comments:	Lots of vegan items in the store, including things to take with you for a quick meal. New location in downtown Summerlin outdoor shopping mall.
Contact:	2101 S. Decatur Blvd., Las Vegas, NV 89102
	(702) 367-0227
	7575 W. Washington Ave., Las Vegas, NV 89128
	(702) 242-8240
	www.traderjoes.com
Hours:	8:00 a.m.–9:00 p.m. (Daily)

Tropical Smoothie Café

Category:	Vegan-Friendly
Price Range:	$
Favorite Eats:	Thai Chick'n Wrap with Beyond Meat
Comments:	Substitute Beyond Meat Chick'n Strips in any wrap, salad, and so on.
Contact:	www.tropicalsmoothiecafe.com

Veggie Delight

Category:	Vegetarian and Vegan-Friendly
Price Range:	$
Favorite Eats:	Crispy Chick'n Sandwich Black Vinegar Chick'n
Comments:	Lots of good vegan options here at Veggie Delight.
Contact:	3504 Wynn Rd., Las Vegas, NV 89103 (702) 310-6565 www.veggiedelight.biz
Hours:	11:00 a.m.–9:00 p.m. (Daily)

Veggie House

Category:	Vegetarian and Vegan
Price Range:	$–$$
Favorite Eats:	Spicy Crispy Beef Kung Pao Chicken Veggie Beef Rolls

Comments:	Chef Kenny is a master with faux meats and flavors. We've needed a place like this, and it is finally here. Some of the best Chinese food, period.
Contact:	5115 Spring Mountain Rd., Las Vegas, NV 89146 (702) 431-5802 www.veggiehousevegas.com
Hours:	11:00 a.m.–9:30 p.m. (Daily)

Vintner Grill

Category:	Vegan-Friendly
Price Range:	$$–$$$
Favorite Eats:	Vegan Portobello Mushroom Picatta
Comments:	Beautiful restaurant in Summerlin. This dish just plain rocks!
Contact:	10100 W. Charleston Blvd. #150, Las Vegas, NV 89135 (702) 214-5590 www.vglasvegas.com
Hours:	Sun–Thurs 11:00 a.m.–10:00 p.m. Fri–Sat 11:00 a.m.–11:00 p.m.

Violette's Vegan Organic Eatery and Juice Bar

Category:	Vegan
Price Range:	$–$$
Favorite Eats:	Red Rock Nachos Samurai Burger Rise 'n Shine Platter

Comments:	Healthy vegan food and a popular location for vegan events and meet-ups.
Contact:	8560 W. Desert Inn Rd., Las Vegas, NV 89119 (702) 685-0466 www.violettesvegan.com
Hours:	Mon–Thurs 11:00 a.m.–9:00 p.m. Fri 11:00 a.m.–10:00 p.m. Sat–Sun 10:00 a.m.–10:00 p.m.

Virgin Cheese

Category:	Vegan
Price Range:	$$
Favorite Eats:	Sriracha Cheddar Smoked Gouda Cheddar "Bacon" Ball
Comments:	Artisanal cashew nut milk–based cheeses produced locally and available at Tivoli fresh52 Farmers' Market on Saturdays and at some local restaurants, including VegeNation and Vintner Grill.
Contact:	www.virgincheese.com

Wahoo's

Category:	Vegan-Friendly
Price Range:	$
Favorite Eats:	Wafu Bowl
Comments:	Nice beach vibe that now has some things vegetarians and vegans will want to eat. Two Westside locations.

Contact:	1000 S. Rampart Blvd., Las Vegas, NV 89145
	(702) 776-7600
	7020 W. Sunset Rd., Las Vegas, NV 89113
	(702) 399-1665
	www.wahoos.com

Whole Foods Market

Category:	Vegan-Friendly
Price Range:	$–$$
Favorite Eats:	Vegan Hot Foods
	Salad Bar
	Taco Bar
	Sandwiches
	Deli Items
	Vegan Pizza
	Baked Goods
Comments:	Great vegan options to eat there or take home with you.
Contact:	8855 W. Charleston Blvd., Las Vegas, NV 89117
	(702) 254-8655
	7250 W. Lake Mead Blvd., Las Vegas, NV 89128
	(702) 942-1500
	www.wholefoodsmarket.com
Hours:	8:00 a.m.–10:00 p.m. (Daily)

Wine 5 Café

Category:	Vegan-Friendly
Price Range:	$–$$
Favorite Eats:	Veggie Delight, Kenyan-Style with Brown Rice

Comments:	African-infused flavors.
Contact:	3250 N. Tenaya Ave., Las Vegas, NV 89129
	(702) 462-9463
	www.wine5cafe.com
Hours:	Mon–Fri 11:00 a.m.–9:00 p.m.
	Sat–Sun 9:00 a.m.–9:00 p.m.

Guidebook Note

All of the information found in this guidebook is based on personal visits made to each restaurant. Restaurants frequently change menu items so some items listed may no longer be available, but they may have comparable new options to try.

It is a good idea to let your server know you are vegan and request that he or she inform you of any ingredients that might not work for you. Most restaurants are very open to working with you and will even create off-menu items to satisfy you. It never hurts to ask questions. You will often be pleasantly surprised by what these people will do for you.

Remember that many servers, and even restaurant owners, are still coming up to a full understanding of what vegetarians and vegans can enjoy, as well as the things that we choose not to. Always be kind and supportive of what they are doing. Remember, we are building bridges and we can do as much for them as they are doing for us.

Please take care of your servers and be the kind of person they will look forward to serving again and again.

That the world is changing is evident from the range of plant-based food options that are before us. We can no longer use the excuse that there are no places for vegans to eat. Enjoy.